ESSAYS ON THE
FIRST HUNDRED YEARS
OF ANAESTHESIA

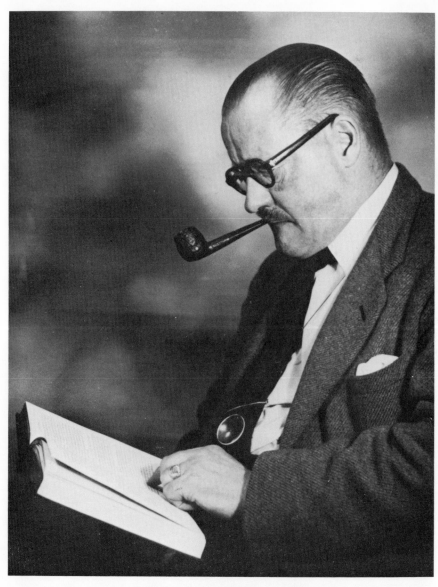

DR. W. STANLEY SYKES
1894–1961

ESSAYS ON THE FIRST HUNDRED YEARS OF ANAESTHESIA

by

W. STANLEY SYKES
M.B.E., M.B., B.Chir.(Cantab.), D.A.

*Late Anaesthetist to the General Infirmary at Leeds, to the Hospital for Women
and St. James' Hospital, Leeds, to the Leeds Dental Hospital, to the
Halifax Royal Infirmary and to the Dewsbury General Hospital*

Volume III

Edited by

Richard H. Ellis
M.B., B.S., D. Obst. R.C.O.G., F.F.A.R.C.S.

*Consultant Anaesthetist to the Royal Hospital of Saint Bartholomew, London
and to The Hackney Hospital, London*

Foreword by

C. Langton Hewer
M.B., B.S., M.R.C.P. (Lond.), F.F.A.R.C.S.

WOOD LIBRARY – MUSEUM OF ANESTHESIOLOGY
Sponsored by
AMERICAN SOCIETY OF ANESTHESIOLOGISTS
515 Busse Highway, Park Ridge, Illinois 60068

CHURCHILL LIVINGSTONE
Medical Division of Longman Group Limited

Distributed in the United States of America and
Canada by the American Society of Anesthesiologists Inc.,
515 Busse Highway, Park Ridge, Illinois 60068. Distributed
elsewhere throughout the world by Churchill Livingstone
and associated companies, branches and representatives.

First published 1982

ISBN 0 443 02865 6

Printed in Great Britain

TO NAN

who pushed me into this labour of Hercules in the first place; and who helped, loved, cherished and over-fed me through the joyous and delightful years of its fulfilment;

AND IN MEMORY OF
MY FATHER

who had a cholecystectomy done by a most skilful surgeon, with all the ritual, panoply, safety and security of modern surgery, . . . and died thereafter.

AND IN MEMORY OF
HER FATHER

to whom exactly the same tragic thing happened.

In the hope that this work may help indirectly towards safer surgery. For the value of history lies in the fact that we learn by it from the mistakes of others. Learning from our own is a slow process.

FOREWORD

Dr. William Stanley Sykes was a very remarkable man. He had a great gift for writing, a passion for accuracy, especially in history, and an excellent grasp of general medicine and anaesthesia.

Dr. Sykes' first book *A Manual of General Medical Practice* was written in 1927 when he was in practice in Morley, near Leeds. He then became interested in anaesthesia, was appointed to the staff of the Leeds General Infirmary and wrote the volume on anaesthesia in the "Modern Treatment" series in 1931.

During the Second World War Dr. Sykes was taken prisoner in Greece, but returned to Leeds after his release. As a perfectionist he became so dissatisfied with the running of the Anaesthetic Department at the Infirmary that he threatened to resign unless things improved. He did, indeed, not only resign, but gave up anaesthesia altogether and returned to general practice.

At this point Dr. Sykes began writing in earnest. He began with three thrillers, one of which *The Missing Moneylender* was issued in the *Penguin* series. He finally embarked on his *magnum opus*, a series of *Essays on The First Hundred Years of Anaesthesia*. The first volume was published in 1960 and the second during the following year, but this occurred after his sudden death at the age of 66.

Volumes I and II were extremely well written and documented: they attained considerable popularity in the United Kingdom and in North America, and were reprinted in the United States in 1972.

It is immediately apparent that Dr. Sykes' account of the early days of chloroform differs radically from that of the Scots surgeons, and he does not hesitate to say so. For example, he comments on an obituary notice of Sir James Y. Simpson in *The Lancet* of the 4th May, 1870 as follows: "This is mostly pure boloney. There are four mistakes in one short paragraph." He then proceeds to enumerate them. The reader will appreciate that this is no dull history, and this explains why the third volume is so eagerly awaited.

The delay in its publication is due to various factors. Dr. Sykes left a vast body of notes which were passed to Dr. de Clive Loewe who, unfortunately, died before he could begin the work. Dr. Bryn Thomas was then asked to prepare the volume for publication and had just started to do so when he also died. Eventually, through the medium of Dr. W. D. A. Smith, of Leeds,

Dr. Richard H. Ellis of St. Bartholomew's Hospital, London, agreed to work on the extremely difficult and onerous task, and has now completed the third volume.

Readers will agree that the delay has been well worthwhile, and that the style typical of Dr. Sykes' previous essays has been continued. Perhaps the rather trenchant passages can best be explained by the fact that he always put the literal truth before the tactful approach. However, readers must judge for themselves.

London, 1982   C. LANGTON HEWER

ACKNOWLEDGEMENTS

First and foremost, the debt which all who have an interest in the history of anaesthesia owe to the late Dr. Stanley Sykes should be recorded. It is well-nigh impossible adequately to express our gratitude for his vision in conceiving such a series of essays, his energy in researching them, and his literary skill in writing them. To most he is a revered name; to a fortunate few he was a colleague and friend; to all he epitomises a diligent seeker after the truth, and one who realised all too clearly that the lessons which can be learnt from history may easily, and with great advantage, be applied to contemporary practice.

I have been helped, as Editor of this Volume, by a great number of people, principal among whom are the following. Mrs. Nancy Sykes, Dr. Sykes' widow, did me a great honour when she allowed me to work on her late husband's papers and prepare them for this publication: she also provided the precious photograph which forms the frontispiece of the book. The late Dr. Bryn Thomas was determined to see the work published and made a number of useful and erudite annotations on Dr. Sykes' typescript. After her husband's death Mrs. Nancy Thomas, knowing of the importance of the papers, made sure that they would be kept safely until the task entrusted to her late husband could be taken over by someone else. Dr. Denis Smith, making light of his many other preoccupations, took up the task of ensuring the continuation of the project, and suggested that I might attempt the work. The American Society of Anesthesiologists, personified by Drs. Charles Tandy and K. Garth Huston, has most generously provided a subsidy to defray the costs of publication of this volume and the simultaneous re-publication of its two, earlier companions. I am most grateful to Dr. C. Langton Hewer for writing the foreword.

The completion of my task would have been impossible without the help of many librarians who have custody of obscure, and often priceless, manuscripts relating to the subjects discussed in the book. Principal among these are the librarians of the Medical College's Libraries at St. Bartholomew's Hospital, London, the Guildhall Library in the City of London, the Libraries of the Royal College of Surgeons of England, the Royal Society of Medicine and the British Medical Association, together with those at the Wellcome Institute for the History of Medicine and the British Library.

Similarly, the work and enthusiasm of a number of photographic departments, and Departments of Medical Illustration has been invaluable. I am especially indebted to Mr. David Tredinnick, and his staff, of the Department of Medical Illustration at St. Bartholomew's Hospital, London, and am grateful to the photographic staff at the Wellcome Institute for the History of Medicine, the Royal Society of Medicine, and the National Hospital for Nervous Diseases in London. Dr. A. H. B. Masson, of Edinburgh, kindly supplied the portrait of Edward Lawrie, and Professor Sykes, of the Nuffield Department of Anaesthetics at Oxford, allowed the reproduction of the two famous illustrations of Joseph Clover at work. The archivist's staff at the Peninsular and Oriental Steam Navigation Company were kind enough to identify the ship on which Lauder Brunton journeyed to India in 1889, and to provide a photograph of the vessel. Similarly, I am grateful to the staff of The India Office Library and Records Department in London who located the portrait of the Nizam and the scenes of Hyderabad in the late nineteenth century. It is a pleasure to record my most sincere thanks to Professor Jean Aubertin and Dr. Charles Laserre, of Bordeaux, France, who located and provided the picture of Dr Oré in Chapter 7. They responded to my plea — that of an absolute stranger — with a vigour and enthusiasm which I think would, hitherto, have been difficult to summon up had our rôles been reversed. A number of publishers have also given permission for the reproduction of illustrations of which the copyright is theirs and, again, I am most grateful for the co-operation.

When I first contemplated the task of editing Dr. Sykes' material I thought that there would not be much more involved than reviewing a manuscript, collating the papers, and sending them off to the publishers. In the event, to be true to my own ideals, and to Dr. Sykes' insistence upon accuracy and truth, an enormous amount of work was needed to scrutinise each reference, to consult other authorities, and to identify that which, with the perspective of history, was not only the real sequence of events but also the correct lesson to be learnt. This was a huge undertaking and I am grateful to all my colleagues at Bart's, senior and junior, who allowed me time during the working days to continue with this task.

I know of no words which can adequately express my gratitude to Elizabeth, my wife, and our three children, Charlotte, Nicolette and Thomas, each of whom shared my enthusiasm for the work, and made considerable sacrifices to see it completed. For their support, optimism, criticisms and laughter I will, eternally, be grateful.

RICHARD H. ELLIS

ILLUSTRATIONS

Figures 2, 3, 4, 5, 12, 13 and 14 are reproduced by kind permission of The Royal Society of Medicine.

Figures 7, 9, 10, 11, 29 and 30 are reproduced by kind permission of the Trustees of the Wellcome Institute for the History of Medicine.

Figures 19, 23, 24, 25, 26, 32, 36, 38, 40, 42, 45, 46 and 75 are reproduced by kind permission of the Editor of *The Lancet*.

Figures 18, 20, 22, 27, 33, 35 and 44 are reproduced by kind permission of the Editor of the *British Medical Journal*.

Figures 66, 67, 69, 72, 73 and 74 are reproduced by kind permission of the India Office Library and Records, London.

CONTENTS

INTRODUCTION

Dr. Sykes retired from the active and clinical practice of anaesthesia at the end of the Second World War, having been held as a prisoner-of-war by the Germans for the preceding four years. Soon after this he began to devote an increasing amount of his time to studying the history of anaesthesia, on which subject he wrote a large number of essays. The first nine were published in 1960 as the first volume of his *Essays on The First Hundred Years of Anaesthesia*: Dr. Sykes prepared a further seventeen essays for publication but died before they appeared in print in 1961. (His fascinating, and highly individual preface to the first volume is well worth reading as a separate essay.) Both volumes were greeted enthusiastically throughout, virtually, the whole of the English-speaking world, and attracted excellent comments from most reviewers at the time. Stanley Sykes' literary style, his wide knowledge of his subject, his level-headed appraisal of the facts, and his ability to make what have been best described as "forthright" statements all combined to produce two books which are treasured by those fortunate enough to possess them, and much sought after by those who do not have copies of their own. The successful, two-volume, facsimile reproductions, which appeared in 1972 attested to the work's continuing popularity. These were published, at the behest of the American Society of Anesthesiologists, by the Robert E. Krieger Publishing Company, of New York.

A study of some of Dr. Sykes' correspondence reveals that he had also worked on material for many more essays on the first hundred years of anaesthesia, and hoped that these would be published as Volumes III, IV and, possibly, V. After his sudden death in 1961, the bulk of this material, together with other papers, old apparatus and his card index of anaesthetic history, went to his friend and former fellow prisoner-of-war Dr. de Clive Loewe in Guildford, where all the material was kept intact. Unfortunately, after Dr. de Clive Loewe's death, in 1977, it was split up; the papers on which this volume is based passed to Dr. Bryn Thomas, in Reading, together with some other papers and the card index. Those papers which Dr. Sykes had hoped would form the basis of Volumes IV and V were not so fortunate and, now, are untraceable. On two occasions in this present volume references are made to these missing essays, firstly on page 24 to an essay entitled *The enquiry before the Senate: one hundred thousand dollars at stake*, and secondly, on page 30 to another entitled *Simpson and the Britannica*. Clearly, had it been possible to publish the full five volumes, each of the later books would have been as fascinating a compendium as were Volumes I and II (and, hopefully, this volume as well).

Dr. Bryn Thomas, then the doyen of British historians of anaesthesia and medicine, began work on the papers for this volume before he died in 1978 and, as can be imagined, his various comments and annotations of Dr. Sykes' typescript have been most helpful in the final preparation of these essays for publication. After Bryn Thomas' death, the papers were carefully kept by his widow, Mrs. Nancy Thomas, who, encouraged by the energy and wisdom of Dr. W. D. A. Smith, of Leeds, made certain that the project to publish this volume did not lapse. Dr. Smith, himself, was the obvious choice to assume the editorship at this stage but was unable to do so because of his many other commitments, particularly the preparation of his detailed and scholarly history of nitrous oxide and oxygen anaesthesia for publication as a single volume, entitled *Under the Influence — A history of nitrous oxide and oxygen anaesthesia*. Dr. Smith took the project under his wing and determined that it should continue. Eventually, after a great deal of patient negotiation with all those who, by now, had become involved — Mrs. Nancy Sykes (whose approval was needed), Mrs. Nancy Thomas (who had custody of the papers), Dr. Charles Tandy and Dr. K. Garth Huston (who arranged for the generous financial contribution made by the American Society of Anesthesiologists towards the costs of publication), and Churchill Livingstone, the publishers of the volume — it was suggested in late 1978 that I should edit the material and prepare it for publication; early in 1980 I was formally asked to do so.

I am very grateful indeed to all those people who were involved in this, and to those who did me the honour of asking me to undertake this precious task. Dr. Sykes was the progenitor of this book, and Dr. Smith its midwife; I am glad to have been able to supervise its birth.

When I received the papers on which this volume is based and read them through it became apparent that, while some of the essays were virtually complete and ready for publication, a number were, probably, not yet in their final form. Each essay, therefore, has been carefully scrutinised, and virtually every reference obtained and studied in detail. As far as possible I have consulted the other sources of information to which Dr. Sykes alluded and have also incorporated a number of other references which, I thought, could shed even more light on the various topics. As a result, some parts of some of the chapters have been re-written, and the construction of a number of the essays has been altered since, by so doing, I thought that the impact of Dr. Sykes' writings would be increased. Similarly, a few of Dr. Sykes' original illustrations have been omitted, and a number of others added.

In making these amendments my over-riding objective has been to ensure historical accuracy. I hope that the various alterations which I have made will not be recognised as such, since my second most important objective has been to preserve Dr. Sykes' own, individual, literary style and approach to his subjects. There are many pitfalls which an editor may encounter while performing such a task, and I have tried to avoid those I have recognised. However, I am very aware that few, if any, latter-day composers have successfully put the final touches to Schubert's *Unfinished Symphony*.

The material which I received amounted to more than enough for one volume but was insufficient for two and, therefore, some selection had to be made. After much thought, I decided not to include five essays which, for the sake of completeness, must be mentioned briefly.

"The revival of nitrous oxide" seems to add little, if anything, to the later, definitive work by Denis Smith on the history of nitrous oxide and oxygen anaesthesia. Similarly, "The chronology of anaesthesia" has much in common with a similar list which appeared in *The Evolution of Anaesthesia* by the late M. H. Armstrong-Davison. "The ignoramus and the patent" consists, almost entirely, of letters and articles written by Dr. W. T. G. Morton and which appeared in *The Lancet* of July 17th, 1847 and the *Boston Medical and Surgical Journal* of September 11th, 1850, together with Morton's application to patent his discovery of ether anaesthesia which was copied in the *Boston Medical and Surgical Journal* on April 7th, 1847. "The very first, deliberate, authenticated use of anaesthesia for surgery in the history of the world" is copied, word for word, from Crawford Long's original article which appeared in 1849 in the December issue of the *Southern Medical and Surgical Journal*. I thought long and hard about one other essay, entitled "The estimation of operative risk", before deciding not to include it in this volume. (By 1935 Dr. Sykes had written articles which dealt, largely, with this subject and which were published in the *British Journal of Anaesthesia* and *Anesthesia and Analgesia: Current Researches*). This essay, I thought, was not at all typical of the others in this or the preceding two volumes and, in the circumstances, I felt justified in leaving it out.

This material will not be lost to future students who may wish to re-assess it. I hope that, eventually, it will be possible to hand over all the working papers used in the preparation of this volume, together with Dr.

Sykes' other papers and his card-index, to a suitable library of historic anaesthetic texts.

London July, 1982   Richard H. Ellis

CHAPTER I

THE RETICENCE OF DR. LONG

I often wondered what possible explanation there could be for the inexplicably secretive behaviour of Dr. Crawford W. Long. He was, beyond question, the first person in the world who deliberately and successfully used ether as an anaesthetic. This was on 30th March, 1842. The long, complicated and rather undignified controversy as to priority between Wells, Morton and Jackson collapsed at once when Crawford Long finally broke silence and produced his evidence some seven years after the event. Even the incorrigible Charles T. Jackson was convinced and took Long's claim up as a means of discrediting Morton.

But why, why did Dr. Long wait for seven years before making his claim to priority of ether anaesthesia?

Obviously, the first step in trying to solve this mystery was to get hold of the writings of the man himself and to read them. It was also necessary to study his life and character as revealed by other people.

Long's famous and classical article appeared in the *Southern Medical Journal*, published in Augusta, Georgia in 1849.[1] I anticipated considerable difficulty in getting a copy of this. After all, the issue in question was well over a hundred years old, and the journal itself was one of local importance only and of small circulation. The population of the whole state of Georgia, at that time, was only half a million, nearly half of whom were slaves. Had any copies survived? The Inter Library Loan system proved equal to the task, however, and produced the required volume, with very little delay, from Manchester University.

After reading Crawford Long's article carefully and copying it out verbatim I still did not know the answer to my own satisfaction. Long's reasons, as given by himself, did not sound very convincing. They were good enough to explain some delay, but not to explain seven years.

The first of his reasons was that he was busily engaged in, and distracted by, the work of a very laborious, country practice. Secondly there were his doubts as to whether he really had priority, and these were strong enough for him to wait until other contestants were in the ring. With his natural modesty he appears to have had the feeling that "It cannot happen to me — a country doctor does not make great, scientific discoveries. The whole thing is impossible." His next reason was his own negligence, and his fourth excuse was that he had had so few opportunities for using ether. In 1842 he had tried his method in only three cases, all of which were successful; by "Ether Day", four years later, he only had a total of eight cases. His fifth reason for the delay in publicising his experiences was that he had been, at first, doubtful whether the effect was due to the ether or whether it was due to imagination, self-hypnosis or to a natural insensibility to pain. He had, as it happened, come across two controlled cases which had satisfied him on this point. One was the amputation of two fingers in a negro slave boy. The first finger he removed with ether and the second without; the contrast between the two episodes impressed him. This case was operated upon on the 8th January, 1845, but I was not able to discover the date of his other controlled observation. Nonetheless, it is fair to assume that a delay until this date was reasonable and justifiable on the grounds of scientific caution. That still leaves unexplained, however, the period from January 1845 until December 1849; nearly five years.

It must be remembered that about this time there were quite a number of isolated cases of painless surgery under hypnotism reported from many parts of the world. The idea of painless surgery itself was just beginning to be accepted, at any rate, by some people; what was not accepted, and not even thought of, was that painless surgery could be achieved by the inhalation of a vapour. Crawford Long said that he did not believe in hypnotism — or mesmerism as it was often called then — and yet there must have been at least a faint shred of doubt in his mind because not until he had a control case was he able to satisfy himself that mesmerism could not possibly have been the reason for his success.

His sixth reason was that he had had no opportunity of using ether for any serious or severe operation. Lastly, he pleaded his isolation. "Had I been engaged in the practice of my profession in a city . . . the discovery would, no doubt, have been confided to others . . ."

My next step was to obtain a copy of Crawford Long's biography, written by his daughter, Mrs. Frances Long Taylor.[2] It is clear that she loved, honoured and revered his memory as a father, as a doctor and as a man. She described him as a Southern gentleman of a vanished day, with a strong sense of the tremendous responsibilities that were his inheritance. These responsibilities included the slaves he owned.

It is not easy for us to enter the minds of those to whom slavery was an accepted routine and normal custom, age-old and immutable. Their thoughts worked differently from ours. Long was a devout Christian but saw, in slavery, nothing that was incompatible with his religion. He believed that the Providence of God permitted it to be in order to christianise the African races, and he regarded his slaves as a sacred trust.

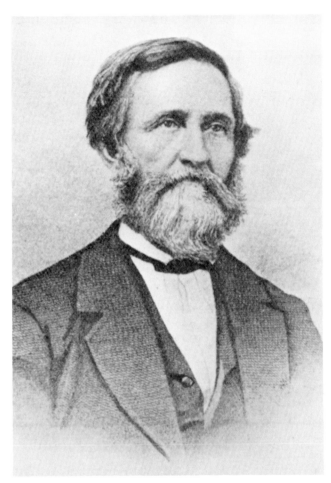

FIGURE 1

Crawford Williamson Long, 1815–1879.
Pioneer of anaesthesia, who made the first, deliberate and authenticated use of ether for surgical anaesthesia. This he did on the 30th March, 1842.

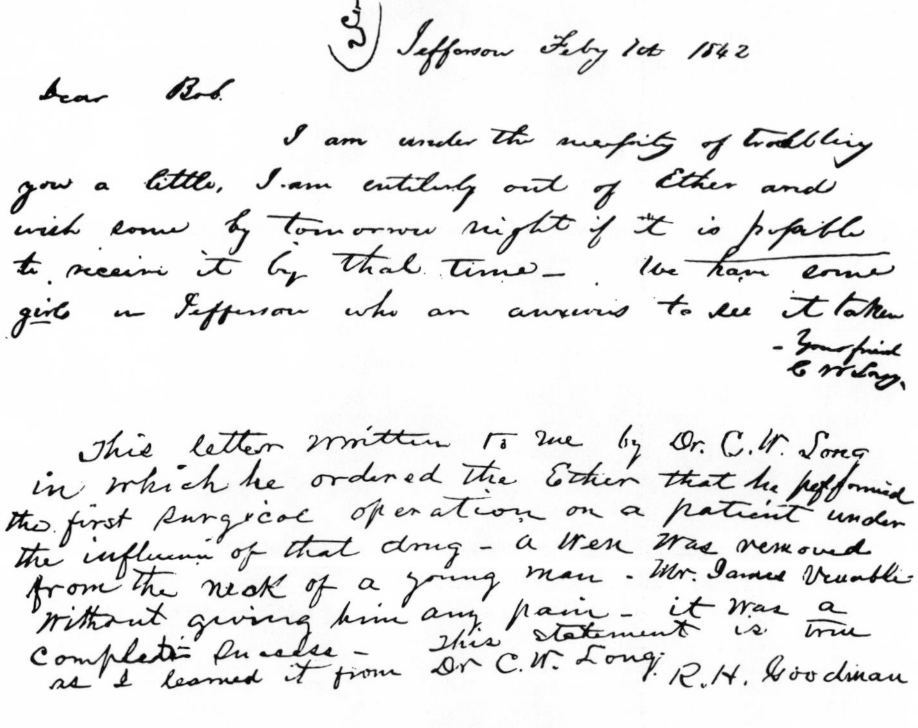

[Handwritten letter]

Jefferson Feby 1st 1842

Dear Bob,

I am under the necessity of troubling you a little, I am entirely out of Ether and wish some by tomorrow night if it is possible to receive it by that time — We have some girls in Jefferson who are anxious to see it taken

— Yours find
C W Long

This letter written to me by Dr. C. W. Long in which he ordered the Ether that he performed the first surgical operation on a patient under the influence of that drug — a Wen was removed from the neck of a young man - Mr. James Venable without giving him any pain - it was a Complete success - this statement is true as I learned it from Dr C. W. Long. R. H. Goodman

FIGURE 2

Crawford Long's letter to his local chemist in which he ordered the ether for the first operation performed under ether anaesthesia — the excision of a tumour from the neck of a young man, named James Venable. Added to this is a letter from the chemist, R. H. Goodman, affirming his belief in Long's priority in the use of ether.

Their work was not especially profitable, but their natural output of babies offered prospects of capital appreciation. Only Dr. Long would never sell them and take his profit — with the exception of one man whom Mrs. Taylor described as a confirmed rogue.

I have no doubt that this man was sold cheaply with his faults pointed out to the buyer, for Dr. Long was utterly and rigidly honest. Just before the beginning of the Civil War he ordered, with considerable foresight, a large stock of drugs from Northern firms, knowing that there would soon be a shortage. The shipment was confiscated as contraband of war by the newly-formed Confederate Government, and Long was obliged to pay them for it. Five years later, at the end of the war during which he had been considerably impoverished, Long paid the bills again, this time to the firms which had originally supplied the drugs. For full measure he added interest to compensate them for the delay. This is a fair testimonial to his iron-clad honesty, whatever the cost to himself personally.

In an age when devaluation of the coinage has become standard practice among the governments of nations, debasement of words has also occurred. The word "gentleman" has suffered in this way and, from being a term of respect, has almost become a term of reproach. But the gentlemen of a century or so ago had their standards and their values and, in many ways, they were high ones. Dr. Long may not have realised the full importance of his discovery at the outset but, when it had become a well-known and accepted fact, he was as anxious as anyone that his claim for priority should be recognised. He would, however, go no farther than this and the idea of making money out of it never entered his head. In a letter to Dr. Paul Eve (then the nestor of Southern surgery) on the 7th March, 1854 which was the day before Charles T. Jackson came to see him, Long wrote:

"I would much prefer my claim to the discovery being admitted by the National Medical Association to any appropriation which might be made by Congress. I am entitled to the credit of priority of discovery, and I am extremely anxious that the honor should be yielded to me by enlightened members of the medical profession."

He had written to his Congressman and to Georgia's Senator, Senator Dawson, about the matter some time previously. The Senator passed the matter over to Dr. Charles Jackson who then visited Long and was, amazingly, satisfied by his evidence. This, I think, was the best possible proof of its strength and authenticity. To convince the pertinaceous and unscrupulous Jackson, whose ruling passion in life appeared to be purloining other people's inventions, was no small feat. But great is truth and strong above all things. No half truths, no pretences and no misrepresentations

5

could prevail against the sworn statements of witnesses, of patients, and the original entries in Long's daybook.

"On taking leave of Dr. Long . . . Dr. Jackson said . . . 'Well, doctor, you have the advantage of us other claimants to the first discovery and use of sulphuric ether as an anaesthetic, but we have the advantage in having first published it to the world'."

On this occasion, if on no other, did Jackson speak the exact and literal truth; but his twisted mind immediately began to work in its usual, tortuous way.

"Jackson proposed to Long to lay their claims conjointly before Congress — he, Jackson, to claim the discovery, and Long to claim the first practical use, his object evidently to get ahead of Morton. This proposition was rejected by Dr. Long, who was satisfied that he was entitled to both.

"On April 15, 1854, the appropriation bill was up before the Senate for its final reading. The friends of Wells and Morton . . . were confidently awaiting the result, when Senator Dawson arose and said that he had a letter from Dr. Jackson which acknowledged that a Dr. Long in Georgia had undoubtedly used ether before any of the claimants.

"Coming as it did from so prominent a contestant, this announcement fell like a thunderbolt on the rival claimants, and from that time they seem to have lost all hope of gaining the reward and passively allowed the bill to die.

"Desirous of preventing another from being recognised by Congress as the discoverer, and not wishing any pecuniary reward himself, Long never pushed the matter further."

He must have known that the proposed reward was one hundred thousand dollars, a nice, large sum by any standard; but the size of it made no difference. Long was not interested.

Before the Civil War Long was prosperous. He had a lucrative practice which meant a great deal of hard work, he owned a drug store, had two plantations worked by slaves which he had inherited, and, above all, he had a happy family life. By this time he had moved from the village of Jefferson to the town of Athens. Then war came. In the non-industrial southern states there were shortages of almost everything, and these grew worse as time passed and the Federal blockade tightened. Formerly rich and still refined families kept up a façade of gracious living, but it was a hollow sham. Negro butlers still served them, but that which was poured from the solid silver coffee pots was a dreadful and inferior liquid made from roots and berries. Old curtains were cut up to make new clothes; money was of little use because the things which money represented were simply not available. In

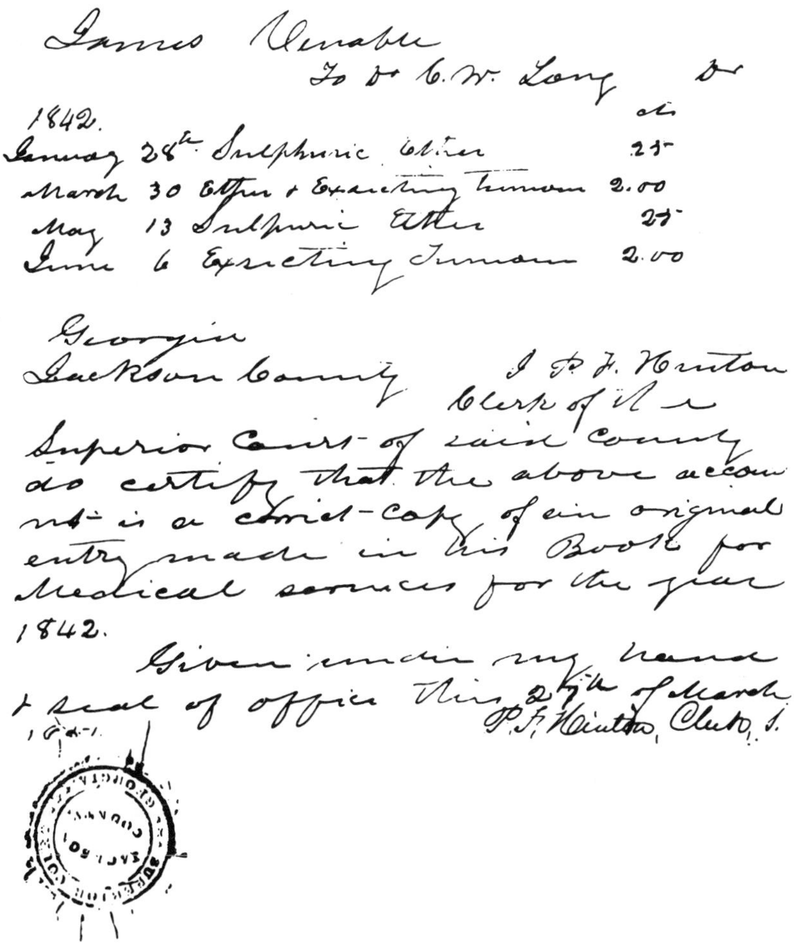

FIGURE 3

A facsimile of Crawford Long's bill, rendered to James Venable, for the first, deliberate and authenticated use of ether for surgical anaesthesia — in 1842.

(Long's fee for the operation and the anaesthesia was 2 dollars. The equivalent 1982 value of this 140-year-old sum is something near 21 dollars (U.S.), or £11·50.)

Below is the much later authentication of the facsimile by the County Clerk of Jackson County, Georgia.

the nineteenth century, poverty was almost a crime but, during this war, it was no disgrace to be poor because everybody was poor. It was only inconvenient and uncomfortable. The men of the households were absent — and many of them never came back; the women had to do the men's work as well as their own. But worse was to come. The Long family, like many others, became refugees, evacuees. They might just as well have been living in the fifth century, fleeing from the onslaught of Attila, or, in the twentieth century in the time of Hitler. I am not suggesting that the Federal troops were deliberately cruel or that they were, in any way, comparable to the two monsters mentioned — but war is never gentle and rarely discriminating.

"One summer morning in 1864, news came that General Stoneman, commanding a division of Federal cavalry, was nearing Athens with orders from General Sherman to burn all the towns and cities . . . take all the mules and horses . . . destroy all provisions and to decoy away all the negroes . . ."

This was a few months before Sherman's famous march through Georgia. Mrs. Frances Taylor was a young girl at the time; she does not state how old she was, nor is her date of birth given in the book. But she does say that she can just remember Dr. Charles T. Jackson's visiting her father in 1854. If she was five years old then — which would be a reasonable guess — she would have been fifteen during the raid.

When the house was abandoned her father entrusted her with a glass jar containing a roll of papers which, he told her "are most important and under no circumstances must be lost, they are the proofs of my discovery of ether anaesthesia." The jar was tied to her waist with rope and her skirt lengthened to conceal it. She was told to bury it if necessary, and this she did. The advancing column of cavalry was captured by the Confederates before they reached Athens, however, so the family returned home. This incident shows the importance which Long, by then, had attached to his discovery and to the precious documents which proved it and which could never be replaced.

The war, and its aftermath, affected Athens severely. Of 1,513 white men and boys in the town and county, 1,300 entered the Army, and nearly half of them were wounded or died. A Federal garrison was stationed there at the end of the war but, in spite of this, conditions remained very bad for many years. The presence of large numbers of people who had recenly been slaves did not help matters. They were now free; free to starve, free to be idle, free to steal. They were not used to freedom. A few people had managed to save their cotton which, therefore, fetched fabulous prices, but

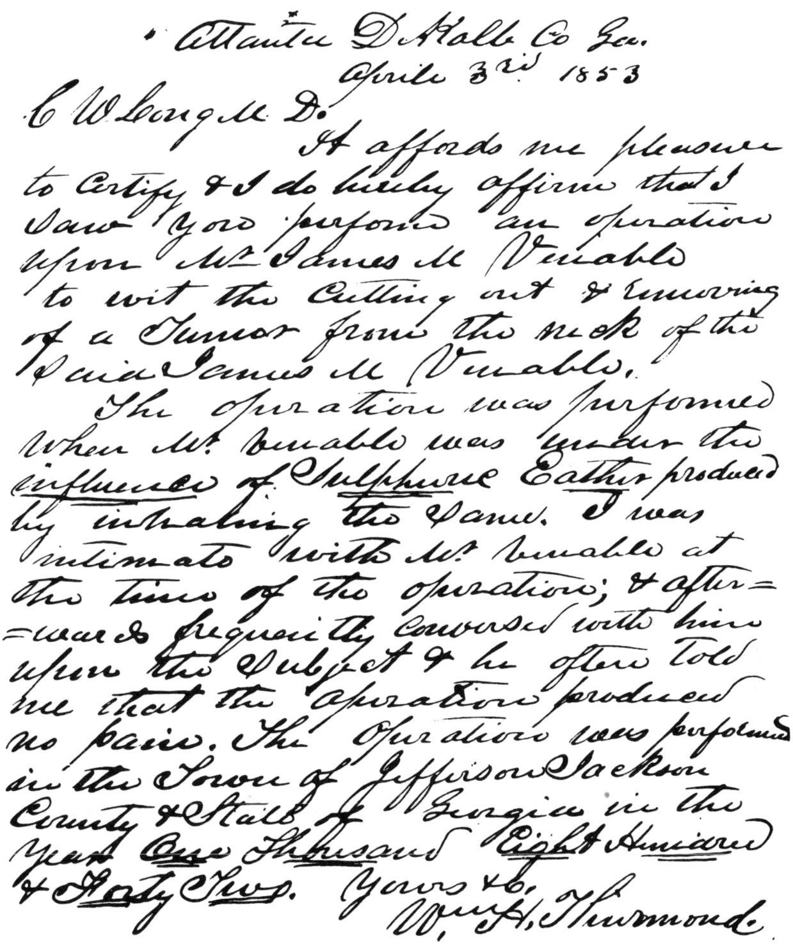

Atlanta DeKalb Co Ga.
April 3rd 1853

C W Long M D

It affords me pleasure to Certify & I do hereby affirm that I saw you perform an operation upon Mr James M Venable to wit the Cutting out & removing of a Tumor from the neck of the said James M Venable.

The operation was performed when Mr Venable was under the influence of Sulphuric Eather produced by inhaling the same. I was intimate with Mr Venable at the time of the operation; & afterwards frequently conversed with him upon the Subject & he often told me that the operation produced no pain. The Operation was performed in the Town of Jefferson Jackson County & State of Georgia in the year One Thousand Eight Hundred & Forty Two. Yours &c.

Wm H. Thurmond.

FIGURE 4

William H. Thurmond was, apparently, present at Long's first use of ether to produce surgical anaesthesia. This is a copy of his certificate, dated April 3rd, 1853, in support of Long's claim to have been the first to have used ether for surgical anaesthesia as we would, nowadays, understand it. For the reasons which I have discussed in the *Essays*, Long did not publicly claim his priority until some seven years later: no-one, to my knowledge, has suggested any reasons why those who are recorded as having witnessed this momentous event remained silent for a somewhat longer period of time.

Dr. Long had, unfortunately, lost eight thousand dollars of it at the time of the raid. The doctor, himself, was treated very well by the garrison, and was even appointed as their chief surgeon — a good example of the beneficent neutrality of Medicine in wartime — a neutrality which has almost always held good, with the awful exceptions of a few Nazi renegades in concentration camps during the Second World War. (Not all German doctors, by any means, were tainted in this way during those hostilities. I was fortunate in meeting only those who upheld the best traditions of Medicine, and treated all men alike. Just as we did.)

Long, again, became prosperous at the cost of much hard work which was to continue to his very end.

"My father's medical responsibilities seemed to grow heavier each day the last few months of his life. He was obliged to leave early in the morning, frequently not returning until late at night. The night before he was seized by his fatal illness we were fortunate in having him with us at supper.... He had never seemed more interested or more cheerful. Finally he grew serious and talked of life and its duties, then rising from the table he said with the greatest gentleness and tenderness: 'No man ever had better children than I have.' This was his farewell to us. When we next saw him he was unconscious."

He went to a confinement, of which he had many, either that night or the next day. After the baby was born he fell forward on to the bed. He was just able to tell the attendant to look after the patient and the baby, but he never spoke again. He was sixty-two years old.

He was not only a gentleman, he was a man; upright, honest, hardworking, incorruptible, devoted to his work and devoted to his family. He once said: "My profession is to me a ministry from God. I am as much called upon to practise Medicine as a minister is to preach the Gospel."

He earned enough to keep his family in comfort and he had some private means; more than that he did not want and would not try to obtain. He desired due recognition, but did not want it paid for in dollars. He was very unlike some of the other claimants. Full and widespread recognition of his priority came only after his death, mainly owing to the efforts of Marion Sims and George Foy. The former had the foresight to persuade Long to have full-length photographs taken which could be, and actually were, used after his death to guide sculptors in the carving of statues of the man.

Crawford Long did his first operation under ether when he was twenty-six years old, less than one year after he had bought Dr. Grant's practice in Jefferson, Georgia.

After reading Mrs. Taylor's account I began to get a clearer idea of the difficulties with which her father had had to contend. The village of Jefferson was 140 miles away from the nearest railway and

"Much of the time in winter the dirt roads were impassable for vehicles, swamps were undrained and streams were forded. A journey of twenty miles was often an all day expedition full of thrills and dangers. . . . Although a young man, he soon acquired a practice which extended for miles into the country."

General practice can be hard work under the best, modern conditions. Even in a built-up area with no great distances to travel, with good roads and a modern car, it can be tiring. How much more so must it have been with the cumulative handicaps of long distances, bad roads and, at best, slow transport. Long's journey by trap or on horseback cannot have averaged more than four miles an hour. There were many confinements, which meant broken sleep and much, weary waiting. A modern doctor, in an urban district, can often fill in the waiting time conveniently by doing other visits nearby; Long, who had to journey for several hours on horseback to reach a labour case at an isolated farm, could not. There he was and there he had to stay until the end, no matter how much work was waiting to be done elsewhere and however long the confinement lasted. Long had no nearby hospital to which he could send his difficult, troublesome or obscure cases; he had no colleagues nearby to consult. Everything had to be done single-handedly.

It is not at all surprising that a man, in these circumstances, found it difficult to write for publication. There just was not time. Long left it on record that he did begin to write up his ether cases on one occasion, but had, very soon, been interrupted by the calls of his practice.

His doubts about priority, which led him to wait until he knew what dates were claimed by the other contenders, were altogether praiseworthy up to a point. But, again, he carried his caution too far and delayed his publication much longer than was necessary. Negligence, of which Long accused himself, probably meant, merely, the combined effects of his other disadvantages — his busy life, his small number of cases and his scientific doubts.

Long had few opportunities of using ether, and this was one of his excuses. He etherised only three patients in 1842, and only a total of eight by the time the discovery burst upon the world four years later. But a few cases were surely enough, in a matter so important and so revolutionary, so utterly and triumphantly new, to have justified publishing them. He would not have needed to make any extravagant claims. He could have, simply and shortly, described his little list of patients and left it to others to try his method for themselves on a larger scale. Busy though he was, this could have been done in a few minutes. He should certainly have done it in January, 1845 when his first case of double finger amputation had removed his doubts about the effects of suggestion and the possibility of self-hypnosis.

His next excuse was that he had had no chance to try ether for any major operation. What difference did that make? The pain of a trivial operation, in those days, was not trivial. If he had published his results ether would have been used soon enough by someone else for more major operations.

He then referred to his isolation in the country. He was isolated but he did meet other doctors occasionally although, according to his daughter, many were sceptical and thought his experiments were dangerous. She wrote that a Dr. Banks, who lived forty miles away, frequently called Long into consultation — yet another example of the demands made upon his time. A journey of eighty miles for such a consultation would have taken at least two days, and probably three, under the conditions as they then were.

As always, many of the lay public were hostile to new ideas.

"He was considered reckless, perhaps mad. It was rumoured . . . that he had a strange medicine by which he could put people to sleep and carve them to pieces without their knowledge. His friends pleaded with him to abandon its use as in case of a fatality he would be . . . lynched. The author knows of but one person who encouraged him by absolute faith, a girl of sixteen to whom he was engaged and who eventually became his wife. The name of the girl was Caroline Swaine."

The small number of his cases was explained, by his daughter, as being due to the placid life of the country. There was "no machinery to mangle people, except the cotton gin, and no other source of accident except runaway horses."

To sum up, Crawford Williamson Long was a modest and unassuming man, who looked upon his profession as a vocation. He was an idealist, with no taint of commercialism. He had the good fortune, and the brains, to introduce something new, but not for a long time did he realise the magnificence of his discovery. Was it likely that an obscure, country doctor could teach something valuable to the expert surgeons of the world? In those early days Long did not, and could not, conceive of the vast increase in surgery to which his work was one of the two contributory factors. As bad luck would have it, he died about the time when Lister was trying to publicise the other factor on which modern surgery depends — the gospel of surgical cleanliness.

It is not given to many men to have the self-confidence of a Morton or a Simpson, especially if they are isolated at the back of beyond and worked to the point of exhaustion in a hard, country practice. The very rarity of Long's operations would tend to lessen the importance of ether in his own eyes, and this is in marked contrast to a busy, town dentist who might have quite a number of small, but painful, operations to perform every day. If you only use something eight times in four years its importance cannot loom very large however well it works and however efficient it is.

Only after the use of ether had been publicised by others, notably by Morton, did the modest and self-effacing country doctor fully realise the tremendous value of the discovery which he had made in 1842. That is my reading of the riddle. That is why Long waited for seven years — because the thing was too incredible and too big.

Crawford Long's own article and his daughter's book about him represent my authorities for this essay. Another reference I consulted was a speech by Thomas J. Collier, of Georgia, in 1942[3] — the centenary year of the first use of ether. There were only two fresh items in it which I had not obtained already. One was that the speaker had, himself, given an anaesthetic to Mrs. Eugenia Long Harper, one of Long's daughters. This was on November 14, 1934 and the patient, aged 73, had a fractured neck of the femur. She lived for six years afterwards. The other item, new to me and of some interest to Scotsmen, was that the speaker referred to Sir J. Y. Simpson of Edinburgh in England. Being a Yorkshireman it is not for me to suggest a suitable revenge.

REFERENCES

[1] Long, C. W. (1849) An account of the first use of Sulphuric Ether by Inhalation as an Anaesthetic in Surgical Operations. *Southern Medical and Surgical Journal*, **5**, 705–713.

[2] Taylor, F. L. (1925) Crawford Williamson Long. *Annals of Medical History*, **7**, 267–296 & 394–424.

[3] Collier, T. J. (1943) Crawford Williamson Long, 1815–1878. *Anesthesiology*, **4**, 279–282.

CHAPTER 2

MORE ABOUT CRAWFORD LONG

Since I wrote the Essay on "The reticence of Dr. Long", and quoted his original description of the very first ether anaesthetic on March 30th, 1842 I have obtained some more information about him. I knew that two accounts of him had been written by Joseph Jacobs, a pharmacist in Atlanta, Georgia who, in his early days, had been apprenticed to Long as surgery-boy and dispensary assistant.[1,2] These, although written at a comparatively late date (in 1919, for Jacobs was much younger than Long) were fairly difficult to get hold of. Finally, however, the Inter Library Loan service obtained them for me from the Library of Congress; both were bound into one small volume.

Much of what Jacobs had to say was already familiar, but there was a good deal of new material as well. Jacobs remembered Crawford Long as a mature and dignified man of middle age, and, like everyone else who had known him, had liked and respected him.

"He was above medium height and wore conventional black. He was quiet and unassuming in deportment and address, gentle and gracious in manner with all whom he conversed, but with ever a retiring and modest mien. He was exacting and particular in business dealings for just and honourable results, and required order, cleanliness and system in all the appointments of the store and office. His kindly disposition and quiet good humor attracted many friends. . . ."

Mrs. Frances Long Taylor, his married daughter, gave a personal description of him to Jacobs, which is not given in her own book:

"He was six feet in height, rather slender when a young man, but in middle life weighed from one hundred and sixty to one hundred and seventy pounds. He was finely proportioned, with broad shoulders, but with small feet and hands, with very thin and tender skin. His forehead was high, broad and full; eyes very blue, well developed nose, somewhat aquiline. Very dignified in manner, his whole appearance betokened the gentleman.

"He maintained a slight reserve, except among intimates and congenial people, or with the sick, absolutely free from all duplicity, never thrusting his opinions upon people, but when expressing them, was frank and fearless. He scorned boastfulness, pretension or any manner of deceit. Cheerful in the sickroom, he always inspired his patients with confidence. His perfect self-control, kindliness and fine judgement gave him great influence, and he was appealed to in many cases to arbitrate.

"Dr. Long dressed well; he generally wore what was called a frock coat. . . . His suits, generally, were made to order by the best tailors, generally of broadcloth. He was particular in all his personal habits. I never knew him go to a meal without first washing his hands.

"He was a very fine whist player . . . fond of hunting* and fishing and was a wonderful shot with the rifle and pistol. . . . As a young man he was fond of dancing, and all of his life, of the theatre and opera, demanding the best acting and music, although he enjoyed a good minstrel show. He had a correct eye for form and taste in colors. . . . His children were trained never to wear imitation jewels or laces. He hated shams of every kind. . . . His was the old-fashioned Southern hospitality. . . . I know of no eccentricities he possessed. He was a singularly well rounded character. He was sensitive, refined and considerate of others; free from envy, malice and all uncharitableness, with quick, high temper, but under control."

He must, indeed, have been a lovable man, sane, sensible, balanced and worthy. Everyone who knew him, everyone who met him, respected him. His widow wrote in 1886, eight years after his death:

"We had prospered in this world's goods, had a lovely home and sweet, pleasant children, two sons and three daughters. My husband was the leading physician, fine-looking, a devoted husband and father, a kind judicious master, beloved and respected by all classes. . . . A large and lucrative practice enabled us to live handsomely, without entrenching on other sources of revenue. . . . Yes, we had an earthly paradise — that of perfect love and harmony. . . . For his dear presence, loving words, fun and frolic, I lived.

"The laborious life of a village doctor, with an extensive practice in the adjoining country and villages and towns without railroads is hard to conceive now. To reach his patients, swollen streams had to be crossed at the fords amid dangers, winter's cold and summer's heat disregarded, with loss of sleep and exhaustion the consequences. . . . His ideals were noble and lofty, causing aspirations to make the most of himself for the good of mankind. For this he loved, labored, suffered and died."

That was the opinion of the person who knew him best of all, who loved him and whose life was shattered when he died.

Long, as I said before, settled first of all in Jefferson, after buying the practice belonging to Dr. Grant. This was in 1841, when he was 25 years old. He moved to Atlanta in 1850 but did not stay there long for, in 1851, he removed again to Athens, still in the same state of Georgia, where he purchased the old drug store in Broad Street. Here he worked with his brother, H. R. J. Long, and with Hal C. Billups, and here Joseph Jacobs joined him as a pharmacy apprentice.

* This would, no doubt, have been hunting in the American sense of the word—what we call shooting.

The latter then gives a list of the memorials which were raised to the memory of the man and his discovery. An oil painting of him was hung in the State Capitol at Atlanta; the state of Georgia chose him as one of the two most celebrated Georgians to be commemorated by statues in the Hall of Fame at Washington, D.C.; a monument was erected as a private gift from a Dr. L. G. Hardman at Jefferson, where Long's first experiments had taken place. A Memorial Hospital for students was named after him at the University of Georgia in Athens, and a bronze medallion was unveiled on the 30th March, 1912, the seventieth anniversary of his first ether anaesthetic, at the University of Pennsylvania from where he had qualified as a doctor. These were some of his rewards.

The second part of Joseph Jacobs' book, *A Distinguished Physician–Pharmacist*, was a reprint of a speech made by the author. It is, largely, a description of the ether controversy, with an appendix of documentary evidence in support of Dr. Long. Eighteen affidavits are given, of varying degrees of importance. First amongst them ranks the sworn statement of James Venable, Long's first ether patient, which was reproduced in full in Long's original article in the *Southern Medical Journal*.[3] Next come certificates from witnesses of this or other operations under ether; one was from Edmund S. Rawls, and James E. Hayes testified to the second operation at which he had been present. There were other testimonials of less direct importance. Sarah Venable, James' mother, said that her son had told her about the wonder of painless surgery soon after his operation had been performed. Philip A. Wilhite swore that in October 1844 he had entered Long's office and continued there for some eighteen months; he had heard about the anaesthetic use of ether soon after his arrival, and swore that it had been common knowledge in the district. Other evidence was even less direct, but all of it pointed in the same direction. Under oath, R. H. Goodman wrote that, in November 1841, Long had told him of his belief that an operation could be performed without pain under ether.

Jos. B. Carlton, M.D. and James Camak, M.D. testified that they had both assisted Dr. R. D. Moore to amputate the leg of a negro boy in May, 1843. Dr. Moore had said, upon his arrival at the case, that, if he had thought of it before leaving home, he would have tried Dr. Long's great ether discovery. This, of course, was some considerable time before Wells and Morton began their experiments with ether.

Some of these affidavits, while not being legally admissible evidence, were of considerable value in confirming the statements of the actual witnesses, and in supporting some of the documentary evidence such as the receipted bill which had been paid by Mr. Venable for the operation.

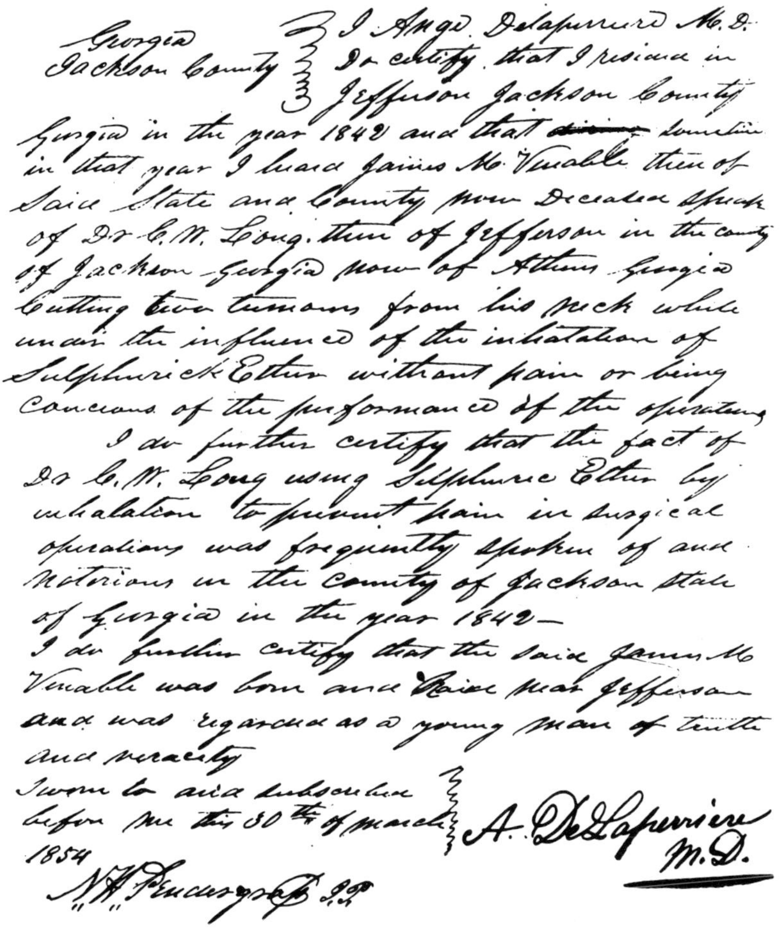
Georgia
Jackson County } I Ango. Delaperriere M.D. Do certify that I resided in Jefferson Jackson County Georgia in the year 1842 and that ~~during~~ sometime in that year I heard James M. Venable then of Said State and County now Deceased Speak of Dr C.W. Long. then of Jefferson in the county of Jackson Georgia now of Athens Georgia Cutting two tumours from his neck while under the influence of the inhalation of Sulphurick Ether without pain or being Concious of the performance of the operation

I do further certify that the fact of Dr C.W. Long using Sulphuric Ether by inhalation to prevent pain in surgical operations was frequently spoken of and notorious in the County of Jackson State of Georgia in the year 1842—

I do further certify that the said James M Venable was born and Raised near Jefferson and was regarded as a young man of truth and veracity

Sworn to and subscribed before me this 30th of march 1854 } A. DeLaperriere M.D.

N.H. Pendergrass J.P.

FIGURE 5

Long's use of ether "by inhalation to prevent pain in surgical operations was frequently spoken of and notorious in the County of Jackson State of Georgia in the year 1842". This letter, dated 30th March, 1854 makes this claim. In 1842, James Venable was at college and so his operation was performed, after he had completed his studies, in the afternoon or early evening of the 30th, March, 1842 (Sims, J. M. 1877 The Discovery of Anaesthesia. *Virginia Medical Monthly*, **4**, 81–100). He would still have been a young man when this letter was written and alluded to his death—"James M. Venable then of said State and County now Deceased". The cause of his death is, at present, unknown, and one can only speculate about whether or not this was in any way connected with the lumps in the neck removed by Dr. Long.

Jacobs also included an account of Dr. Charles T. Jackson's visit to Crawford Long in March, 1854 which followed Long's own claim for precedence which he had put before his State Senator. Amazingly, during this visit Long succeeded in the well-nigh impossible task of convincing Jackson that his claim was genuine. Bearing in mind Jackson's own and determined self-interest in the subject this feat goes a long way to prove that Crawford Long's evidence was watertight and absolutely convincing.

C. H. Andrews, the principal clerk and book-keeper at Long's drugstore, began his reminiscence with a tribute to his famed employer.

"He was . . . patient, gentle and painstaking in fitting me for the struggle and business of life, and I was attentive, anxious to please and ambitious to learn. . . . On March 8, 1854, early in the day, a stranger entered the old drug store in Athens . . . and inquired for Dr. Long. . . . In a few minutes Dr. Long came in, and I said 'This gentleman has come to see you.' The stranger presented his card, introducing himself as Dr. Charles T. Jackson of Boston, Mass."

The famous Dr. Jackson was a "spare made" man, angular, five feet ten inches in height, of swarthy complexion, with dark hair and eyes, and some forty years of age. He was born in 1805, and so was forty-eight when he first met Crawford Long. Andrews described the interview, which ended when Jackson, at Long's suggestion, went to Jefferson to collect evidence at the place where the whole thing began. Two days later, Jackson returned for another long interview with Long.

Jackson gave his own account of his visit to meet Crawford Long in the *Boston Medical and Surgical Journal*.[4]

"Mr. Editor:
"At the request of the Hon. Mr. Dawson, U.S. Senator for Georgia, on March 8, 1854, I called upon Dr. C. W. Long, of Athens, Ga., while on my way to the Dahlonega Gold Mines, and examined Dr. Long's evidence on which his claims to the first practical use of ether in surgical operations were founded, and wrote, as requested by Mr. Dawson, who was then in the United States Senate, all that I learnt on the subject.

"From the documents shown to me by Dr. Long it appeared that he used sulphuric ether as an anaesthetic agent:

"1. On March 30, 1842, when he excised a tumor from the neck of James Venable, a boy in Jefferson, Jackson Co., Ga., now dead.

"2. July 3, 1842, in the amputation of a toe of a negro boy belonging to Mrs Hemphill of Jackson Co., Ga.

"3. September 9, 1843, in the amputation of a tumor from the head of Mary Vinson of Jefferson, Ga.

18

"4. January 8, 1845, in the amputation of a finger of a negro boy belonging to Ralph Bailey of Jackson Co., Ga.

"Copies and depositions proving these operations with ether were all shown to me by Dr. Long, who stated to me that his account book, with the original entries and charges, was in the hands of his attorney at Jefferson, his former residence, for the purpose of having his dues collected, and that he would show me the book when I visited Athens at a future day. He also referred me to physicians in Jefferson who knew of the operations at the time. I then called upon Professors Joseph and John Le Conte, then at the University of Georgia at Athens, and inquired if they knew Dr. Long, and what his character was for truth and veracity. They both assured me that they knew him well and that no one who knew him would doubt his word and that he was an honorable man in all respects.

"Subsequently on revisiting Athens Dr. Long showed me his Folio Journal, or account book, in which stand the following entries:

March 30, 1842	— Ether and excising tumor	$2.00
May 13, 1843	— Sulphuric ether	.25
June 6, 1842	— Excising tumor	2.00

"On the upper half of the same page are several charges for ether sold to the teacher of the Jefferson Academy, which Dr. Long told me was used by the teacher in exhibiting its exhilarating effects, and he said that the boys used it for the same purpose in the Academy. I observed that these records bore the appearances of old and original entries in the book. Of that I have no doubt. The only question is, was the ether thus charged to Mr. Venable employed by inhalation for the purpose of preventing pain and was it actually so used in the surgical operation charged at the time?

"The proofs of this must be in the statement of Dr. Long supported by the affidavit of the parties on whom the operations were performed or who witnessed them. These documents as above stated I have seen in the hands of Dr. Long, or rather copies of them, for the originals were sent to Dr. Paul F. Eve of Augusta, Ga., and were lost by him, so they do not appear in the *Southern Medical Journal* then published by that gentleman.

"On asking Dr. Long why he did not write to me or make known what he had done, he said when he saw my dates he perceived I had made the discovery before him and he did not suppose anything done after that would be considered of much importance, and that he was awakened to the importance of asserting his claims to the first surgical use of ether in operations by learning that such claims were set up by others, and consequently wrote to the Georgia delegation in Congress stating the facts which Senator Dawson requested me to inquire into."

What Dr. Long actually said in his first account of the operations, as one of his reasons for delaying publication, was that he waited until other claimants gave their dates in order to see whether his own really had precedence. When he was convinced of this, and not until then, he published his article.

Jackson's explanation, recorded in the *Boston Medical and Surgical Journal*, sounds to me as though his obsession that he was the discoverer of ether anaesthesia was, once more, coming to the surface having, previously, been suppressed by a cold deluge of contrary fact.

The story that the original papers had been lost is also unlikely to be true. Some, but not all, of the evidence was printed in the original account, and no mention of the loss of any documents is made by the Editor, by Long himself, by his daughter or by Jacobs. The tremendous importance and irreplaceability of these papers was fully realised by Long himself, and to this their secret burial for safety during the cavalry raid in the Civil War, years later, must testify. Jackson continued:

"I have waited expecting Dr. Long to publish his statements and evidences in full and have, therefore, not published what I learned from him. He is a very modest and retiring man, and not disposed to bring his claims before any but a medical or scientific tribunal. This he has done in the State Medical Society of Georgia as appears by their records.*

"Had he written to me in season I would have presented his claims to the Academy of Science in France, but he allowed his case to go by default, and the Academy knew no more of ether in surgical operations than I did.

Boston, April 3, 1861

(sig.) Charles T. Jackson, M.D."

Crawford Long's evidence must, indeed, have impressed Jackson. For years he had been claiming the discovery for himself and had battled against Morton in a most vindictive and vituperative manner. But now, for once, his scientific mind had recognised, absolutely, the watertight and unbreakable evidence with which it had been presented; so impressive was this that he allowed it, for a time, to overcome his own mania for purloining the inventions of other men. Only once in his account does Jackson's *idée fixe* appear. Most of his letter is factual.

Hugh. H. Young, an Assistant Resident Surgeon at Johns Hopkins Hospital in Baltimore, wrote a booklet entitled *Long, the Discoverer of Anaesthesia*.[5] In this he says:

"The list of operations as given by Dr. Jackson is not complete, as he has omitted the second operation on Venable, and a number of the later operations. In a letter to Dr. Sims, which I have, Dr. Long denies absolutely that he ever

---

* See *Southern Medical and Surgical Journal*, Augusta, Ga.

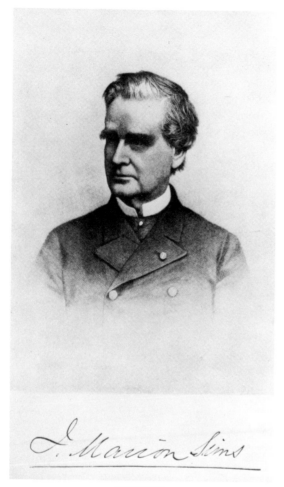

FIGURE 6

Dr. J. Marion Sims. He "championed Long's cause, but unfortunately, his communication, so well conceived, was hurriedly executed and introduced the inaccurate statement that S. C. Wilhite* had suggested to Long the idea of using ether. Wilhite himself contradicted this; as a matter of fact he did not come to live with Long as a student until 1844". (Buxton, D. W. 1912 Crawford Williamson Long (1815–1879): the Pioneer of Anaesthesia and the first to suggest and employ Ether Inhalation during Surgical Operations. *Proceedings of the Royal Society of Medicine*, **5**, i, 19–45.)

* In turn, Dr. Buxton's account is somewhat inaccurate—it was Dr. P. A. Wilhite, of Anderson, S.C. who consulted Long.

acknowledged that Dr. Jackson was the prior discoverer. He had been led to infer that ether had anaesthetic powers several months before he got a chance to verify it, and before Jackson claims to have made similar inferences, but he dated his claims of discovery from the time of his first practical demonstrations. Before that it was a mere supposition, as was Jackson's also.

"But, barring these inaccuracies, Dr. Jackson's paper, coming as it does from one who so zealously coveted the title of discoverer, is a remarkable admission.

"The interview between Long and Jackson must have been most amicable, and Long evidently felt the greatest respect for Jackson. . . ."

If one has to choose between conflicting statements by Long and by Jackson there is no doubt whatsoever who was the more reliable witness. The modest and upright Crawford Long was incapable of telling a lie and was, equally, unlikely to stretch or manipulate evidence to his own advantage. Money meant little to him, and nothing at all when compared to his own honour and his own conscience. Jackson's conduct, throughout, was far more open to suspicion. He was grasping and unscrupulous, a man who did not hestitate to twist the facts to his own advantage whenever this was possible: he was obsessed with his efforts to denigrate Morton.

Jacobs finished his account by quoting a letter from Crawford Long to Charles T. Jackson, which was written eight months after the latter's visit to Georgia, in which Long said that he was writing an article about his claims and that he did not wish to say in it anything which displeased Jackson. He asked for permission to quote Jackson's own admissions, but said that he would not do so without his consent. This, again, shows Long's habitual and meticulous courtesy and also his total inability to take any unfair advantage.

Jacobs, however, did not remain content with giving a wholly one-sided account of the controversy over ether's introduction as an anaesthetic. He quoted an affidavit by H. J. Payne, a surgeon-dentist of Troy, New York, which was dated April 12th, 1848. It was published, with others, by Messrs. Lord and Lord who were Dr. Charles T. Jackson's attorneys.

"On the second day of January, 1847, I went to Boston and sought an interview with Dr. Morton. . . . Dr. Morton stated emphatically and repeatedly that Dr. Charles T. Jackson of Boston was the sole discoverer of the new drug for producing insensibility to pain, and that Dr. Jackson communicated it to him. Furthermore, that all the knowledge he possessed in relation to its properties and application had come to him from Dr. Jackson, and that he never had any idea of applying sulphuric ether, or that sulphuric ether could be applied for the aforesaid purposes, until Dr. Jackson suggested it to him, and had given him full instructions."

I must say that I view any evidence produced by Messrs. Lord and Lord with considerable suspicion. It will be seen in another Essay[6] that sworn evidence was given at the Congress Enquiry by three different witnesses, two dentists and a druggist, to the effect that Mr. Lord had tried to trick them into giving false dates, that he had asked them confusing and misleading questions and that he had even suggested bribes for false statements which they had refused to sign. None of these witnesses had any apparent object to gain by perjury.

Moreover, the above affidavit is in sharp conflict with the admitted facts—that Morton used ether at his own house on Eben Frost, that Morton gave ether to Gilbert Abbott at the Massachusetts General Hospital a fortnight or so later, and continued to give it to other cases until late in November, wholly on his own responsibility and in the absence of Dr. Jackson who never even saw an anaesthetic given until November 21st, 1846. It was Morton who had the practical experience, not Jackson. Consequently, to say that Jackson gave Morton full instructions is quite meaningless. Jackson could, and may, have suggested ether to Morton, although this is by no means certain. If he did do so then he deserves as much credit as does David Waldie, who suggested the use of chloroform to James Simpson. But Waldie, although he was disgruntled — with good reason — at the small acknowledgement he subsequently received from Simpson for his help, never claimed any more than this. He did not pretend that he had given Simpson full instructions about its use which is surely true, since neither, at the time, had tried the agent.

Here, then, is one of the differences between a good story and a bad one. Long's claim, unlike that of Dr. Charles Jackson, had no weak points. Every link of the chain was unbreakable.

REFERENCES

[1] Jacobs, J. (1919) *Some personal recollections and private correspondence of Dr. Crawford Williamson Long, Discoverer of Anaesthesia with sulphuric ether, together with documentary proofs of his priority in this wonderful discovery.* Atlanta, Ga.

[2] Jacobs, J. (1919) *A distinguished physician-pharmacist.* Atlanta, Ga.

[3] Long, C. W. (1849) An account of the first use of Sulphuric Ether as an Anaesthetic in Surgical Operations. *Southern Medical and Surgical Journal,* **5,** 705–713.

[4] Jackson, C. T. (1861). First practical use of ether in surgical operations. Boston Medical and Surgical Journal, **64,** 229–231.

[5] Young, H. H. (1897) Long. The Discoverer of Anaesthesia. A presentation of his original documents. *Johns Hopkins Hospital Bulletin,* **8,** 174–184.

[6] These Essays. *The Enquiry before the Senate : One hundred thousand dollars at stake.**

* This essay is one of those the script of which no longer exists.

CHAPTER 3

HENRY JACOB BIGELOW (1818–1890)

Two interesting books about Dr. Henry J. Bigelow were published in 1900. One was an account of his life,[1] and the other was a reprinted collection of articles written by him and originally published in 1848.[2]

Henry Jacob Bigelow had a great deal to do with the introduction of anaesthesia into medical practice. He was born on March 11th, 1818. His father was Jacob Bigelow who rose to become a senior and influential member of the staff at the Massachusetts General Hospital. Henry Bigelow later joined his father on the staff of the hospital, having qualified as a doctor in 1841. After qualifying, he spent a lot of his time travelling and working in other centres, particularly in Paris, and it was not until 1844 that he started in practice on his own account. He was appointed as Visiting Surgeon to the Massachusetts General Hospital on the 28th January, 1846 but, because of structural alterations and enlargement of the buildings, was not able to begin his work there until late in 1846.

This meant that the beginning of his surgical career coincided almost exactly with the beginnings of ether anaesthesia. Henry Bigelow was a man of vision and imagination, and was a very strong supporter not only of ether anaesthesia itself, but also of Morton's claim to be the discoverer. The vivid impression made on him by Morton's invention and first public demonstration of ether at the Massachusetts General Hospital on Friday, October 16th, 1846 never left him. He wrote:

"Would surgeons have given a surgical dose of ether vapour, on all the existing evidence, five minutes before Morton's successful experiment? . . . It was assuredly difficult enough to persuade them to do so afterwards . . . the first perfect knowledge as to the points of safety, certainty and completeness came through Morton alone."

Next, Bigelow made a prophecy which turned out to be quite correct:

"Many may have been the real discoverers of ether insensibility to pain, and at a remote period. But if so, they have kept it to themselves; . . . Dr. Morton was, according to the evidence in print, both the prime mover and the immediate agent in the introduction of this discovery to the world."

Bigelow made this prophecy in 1848 in an original article which appeared in the *Boston Medical and Surgical Journal*.[3] Four years later, Crawford Long came forward with proof that he had done precisely what

Bigelow had foretold — that is, used ether as an anaesthetic in 1842, but kept it to himself. Bigelow continued:

"Sydney Smith says, in the *Edinburgh Review*, 'He is not the inventor who first says the thing, but he who says it so long, loud and clear that he compels mankind to listen to him'."

and this is what Morton undoubtedly did. Even the undignified controversy as to who should claim priority for the invention of ether anaesthesia had its uses in this respect.

Bigelow went on to produce evidence to the effect that anaesthesia met with stiff opposition in some quarters, and this made it all the more important that it should be loudly, long and clearly proclaimed.

"The *New Orleans Medical Journal* says in the same month (January 1847) 'That the leading surgeons of Boston could be captivated by such an invention as this (the use of ether) excites our amazement. Why, mesmerism, which is repudiated by the *savans* [their spelling, not mine] of Boston, has done a thousand times greater wonders'."

and, to give another example,

"In November, 1847, more than a year after the discovery, we find it stated that in one of the largest hospitals in North America, ether has not been tried at all."

Bigelow then described the stages of anaesthesia, and described them well. He went on to mention the difficulties presented by certain operations.

"Hare lip. With this operation may be included others upon the nose, mouth, fauces and trachea. . . . An operation in this region is often a dissection, and of the parts concerned in inhalation. It is, therefore, impossible to continue etherization during manipulation. If, then, the patient is to remain insensible the surgeon has only the alternative either of profoundly narcotizing the patient in the first instance, or of readministering the ether, often at an inconvenient moment, and when the operation is materially interfered with. Of these courses, the former seems to me to be the least objectionable."

The patient should, Bigelow suggested, be made to lean forward and any blood tending to run back prevented from doing so with sponges. "Protracted operations upon the fauces are difficult, if not impossible, with the use of ether."

He then considered the question of resuscitation. Fresh air, artificial respiration, cold water, galvanism and hot tea or coffee were the methods he recommended.

He mentioned the Winlaton case, and that of Mrs. Simmons in

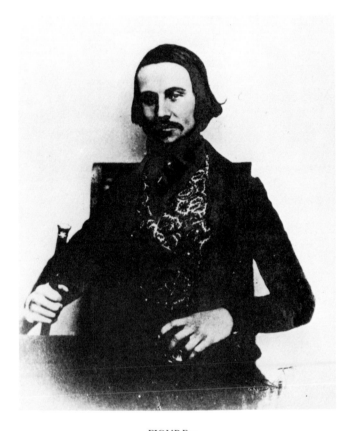

FIGURE 7

Henry Jacob Bigelow in 1841, just 6 years or so before he witnessed Morton's first public demonstration of ether anaesthesia at the Massachusetts General Hospital on 16th October, 1846.

There are several classical illustrations of this momentous event, in each of which both Bigelow and Morton are depicted as being much older than they actually were at the time (Bigelow was aged 29 and Morton was 27). The classical pictures were, almost certainly, later re-creations of the historic scene.

Cincinnati, which were the only two deaths under chloroform given for surgical purposes of which he was aware at the time he wrote. There had been two others, but these could not fairly be debited to chloroform's account. One of them was a druggist's assistant who was in the habit of inhaling it, and who finally gave himself an overdose; he was found with his face buried in a towel on the counter, dead. The other was Horace Wells, who inhaled chloroform before committing suicide by cutting his femoral artery.

Bigelow, like John Collins Warren, was unreliable about dates, for he states that "the date of the announcement of ether anaesthesia is October 1, 1846". (It may, I suppose, have been careless proof-reading after his death.)

He was responsible for the introduction of at least two substances which were tried as anaesthetics. In July, 1861 he reported the use of Kerosolene by inhalation; he had used it in three cases, during one of which a change had to be made to ether. He was first led to try this agent after a man cleaning a tank at a kerosene works had been overcome by it. In April, 1866 he used Rhigolene which was a petroleum naphtha product with a boiling point of 70°Fahrenheit. This he found to be rapid and effective as a freezing agent when sprayed on to the skin.

Bigelow also re-investigated nitrous oxide and concluded that the small bag without valves used by Horace Wells was inefficient and unreliable because of the variable amount of dilution of the gas caused by rebreathing. He considered it suitable only for the gas frolics for which it had been designed. He also suggested the correct explanation for the lividity caused by nitrous oxide anaesthesia — that the gas was a true chemical compound and not merely a mixture which contained as much, or more, oxygen than air. On April 27th, 1848, he used nitrous oxide for the removal of a breast "only eighteen months after the original discovery of practical anaesthesia by ether in November, 1846". This carelessness about dates constantly crops up in his writings.

As the leading surgeon of his day in Boston, Bigelow gave an address at the dedication of the ether monument erected in that city in 1868. He also replied to a letter which Sir James Simpson had written to Professor Jacob Bigelow, his father, in 1870. His father was away at the time. Henry Bigelow was a little unfair in his opinion on this occasion.

"It will be seen that Sir James Y. Simpson considers the introduction of chloroform and its substitution for ether to have been on the whole the most important and culminating event in the history of modern anaesthesia."

Jacob Bigelow had, in fact, attacked Simpson on the grounds that he claimed far too much credit for what he had done — that he almost arrogated the whole discovery of anaesthesia.[4] There was a certain amount of justification for this criticism of Simpson but, unfortunately, the Bigelows had seized upon an incident in which Sir James was entirely blameless of this offence. Simpson was not slow to point this out, and wrote in the next issue of the *Medical Times and Gazette* to explain the circumstances.[5] (The matter is to be fully dealt with in another essay entitled "Simpson and the Britannica".*)

Simpson pointed out, reasonably enough, that the speech referred to was delivered by him on the occasion of his receiving the Freedom of the City of Edinburgh. He, clearly, had had to mention chloroform in his address since that was the part of his work which was best known to the lay public. However, a ceremony honouring an individual by the granting of a city's Freedom was a strictly personal thing and was neither the time nor the place to recount the whole of the history of anaesthesia. Simpson's attitude was, of course, quite correct.

Bigelow then pointed out the most important difference between ether and chloroform — the fact that the former always gave warning of impending danger, while the latter did not. He stated that the records of the Massachusetts General Hospital showed that (in November, 1893) ether had been used in 15,000 cases, of which 6,000 had been in the previous five years. By that time 2,800 pounds weight of ether had been used without a single fatality.

He described the various ways in which the unstable Horace Wells made a living after he gave up the practice of dentistry. He started a business for the sale of patent shower-baths, and he began to buy copies of pictures in the Louvre painted in Paris to be framed and sold in North America. These were both quite legal occupations, but somewhat unusual and eccentric for a dentist.

On the subject of the controversy between Morton and Jackson about the priority of the discovery of ether anaesthesia Henry Bigelow brought out one point which I have not seen mentioned elsewhere.

"The surgeons of the Massachusetts General Hospital, who had no interest whatever in the difference, and could have none, were friends of Jackson, and strangers to Morton. They yielded, when it became necessary to take sides, only to their deliberate conviction of the justice of Morton's claims."

This is an argument of some weight, because the hospital staff were the people who were in the best position to know the facts. The presentation

---

* This essay is one of those the script of which no longer exists.

casket, containing 1,000 dollars in cash and which was given to Morton on the 12th May, 1848, also showed what the Trustees of the hospital thought about the matter.

The *Memoir* of Henry Bigelow gives us some glimpses of the man himself.

"Dr. Bigelow had the faculty of instant decision. He knew every phase of anaesthesia, and if emergencies arose he was prepared for them. Thus in a case of perilous asphyxia from blood entering the trachea during an operation, the ordinary measures of relief under such circumstances having failed, he opened the windpipe with one stroke of a scalpel, passed an elastic catheter beyond the point of obstruction, and blowing through it expelled the clot by driving it upward; the operation then went on. This original method, adopted on the spur of the moment, was first resorted to in June 1867, and has proved equally succesful in similar critical emergencies."

He held very clear-cut opinions, as befitted a person whose active professional life began at the birth of anaesthesia. He had not acquired the protective coat of hard-heartedness, ruthlessness and brutality with which the previous generation of surgeons had to cover themselves in order to do their work at all. He often said "Dying is nothing, but pain is a very serious matter." In 1871 he wrote:

"In a practice of twenty five years I have never intentionally given a patient, unless by his own choice, any pain without narcotization; nor have I allowed a patient to die a painful death when opium would lull him into his long sleep. I share the responsibility of this with the surgeon who walked about the battlefield distributing morphine to those who were hopelessly wounded, and with the soldier, mentioned by Ambroise Paré, who did more."

In one case Bigelow gave a young woman, who was twenty years old and slowly dying from an inoperable sarcoma of her leg, 2,024 grains (121,440 milligrams) of morphine in five weeks — an average of 58 grains (3,480 milligrams) a day. The largest single dose was 120 grains (7,200 milligrams) and at one stage 180 grains (10,800 milligrams) were given in two doses within forty minutes.

An anonymous author once wrote these lines:

> "Friend and physician, in yon little case,
> So poorly hidden in your palm, abides
> That sweet and sleepy essence of the East,
> The master-key of Peace; the which who wields
> Is lord of death."[6]

In the best sense of the word this handsome, fashionable, merciful man was lord of death. His life was happy, successful and hard-working. He was brought up in very comfortable, if not wealthy, circumstances and never had to fight against poverty. His way was made easy for him in that his father had been an eminent member of the hospital's staff before him, but this did not affect his enthusiasm or capacity for work. He did original work on dislocations and on lithotrity — a ligament, a lithotrite and a bladder evacuator are still known by his name. He made his own lithotrites, or at any rate models for them. The only tragic thing about his life was that, as W. J. Mayo once said, "Asepsis and antisepsis came too late for him". He died on October 30th, 1890 in his seventy-second year.

Though he was not an actual pioneer of anaesthesia he helped its early progress enormously. Not only did his receptive mind welcome it enthusiastically and immediately, but he did his best to spread the good news. He wrote the first professional paper on the subject, and it was a reprint of this article which bore the news to England, in the first place, sent by his father in a letter to Dr. Francis Boott.[7]

His influence was felt again at a later date, once more in England, for J. Warrington Haward stated in 1872:

"For more than two years past (owing greatly to the representations of Dr. Bigelow) I have been in the habit of giving ether largely both in public and private practice ... and ... have administered it for the majority of the operations at St. George's Hospital during that period."[8]

This was written before the visit of Joy Jeffries which did so much to reinstate ether in the position which it should never have lost.[9] Haward was one of the very few who used ether in England in 1872 — and he reintroduced it, *pace* Joy Jeffries.

REFERENCES

[1] Anonymous (1900) *A memoir of Henry Jacob Bigelow*. Boston, Little, Brown and Company.
[2] Bigelow, H. J. (1900) *Surgical Anaesthesia. Addresses and other papers*. Boston, Little, Brown and Company.
[3] Bigelow, H. J. (1848) Etherization, a compendium of its history, surgical use, dangers and discovery. *Boston Medical and Surgical Journal*, 229–245, and 254–266.
[4] Annotation. (1870) Sir James Simpson and the late Dr. Morton. *Medical Times and Gazette*, **1**, 67–68.
[5] Simpson, J. Y. (1870) Historical letter on the introduction of anaesthetics in dentistry and surgery in America, and on their first employment in midwifery in Great Britain. *Medical Times and Gazette*, **1**, 90–91.
[6] "Tertius" (1903) Epistle of Ariadne to Theseus. *St. Bartholomew's Hospital Journal*, **10**, 135.
[7] Boott, F. (1847) Surgical operations performed during insensibility. *Lancet* **1**, 5–8.
[8] Haward, J. W. (1872) Ether v. chloroform. *British Medical Journal*, **2**, 534–535.
[9] Editorial. (1872) Ether v. chloroform. *British Medical Journal*, **2**, 499–501.

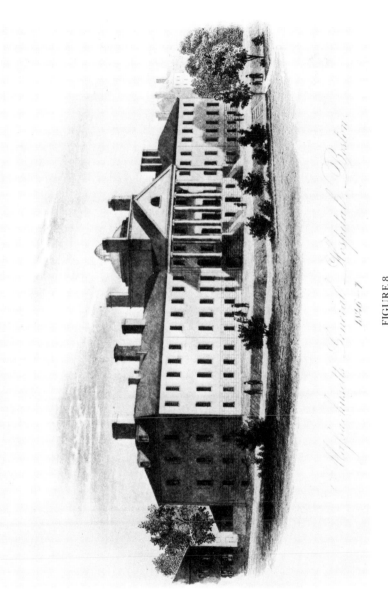

FIGURE 8

The Massachusetts General Hospital as it appeared in 1846. The ether dome, almost the highest point of the building, can be seen clearly. Morton arrived late for his first public demonstration of his "Letheon" before the assembled staff of the Hospital, and must have been apprehensive as he walked up the several flights of stairs to the operating theatre. Had he known how successful his demonstration was going to be he would have been confidence itself. "Before October 16, 1846, surgical anaesthesia did not exist — within a few months it became a world-wide procedure. . . . In science the credit goes to the man who convinces the world, not to the man to whom the idea first occurs. Morton convinced the world: the credit is his." (W. Osler (1917) The first printed documents relating to modern surgical anaesthesia. *Annals of Medical History*, **I**, 329–332.)

CHAPTER 4

WHAT'S IN A NAME?

James Young Simpson signed all his writings in that manner, or in the shortened form "J. Y. Simpson". It had never entered my head to doubt his name, for few are better known than his in the long history of Medicine, and nowhere in print during the whole of my "hundred years" did I find any uncertainty expressed by anyone. It would seem as unreasonable to doubt the name of Julius Caesar, or to say that the Emperor Napoleon's name was not Bonaparte.

A rumour, however, came to my notice from two sources. The first was while I was speaking with a Highland Scot who had heard one of his lecturers at St. Andrews say that Sir James was never christened "Young" at all, but adopted this name in later life. The second was in 1960; in an article Dr. Armstrong Davison, of Newcastle, mentioned (rather vaguely) the same rumour and worded things in such a way as to imply that his readers would know all about it.[1] At the time, I was corresponding with Dr. Armstrong Davison on another historical anaesthetic point and so I told him that I, myself, did not know how accurate the story was, and mentioned that I had heard it spoken of only once before and had never seen it anywhere in print until I read his paper. He replied that Simpson had been rather conscious of his age — or lack of it — when he applied for the Chair of Midwifery at Edinburgh in 1839 and, perhaps in a spirit of bravado, had called himself James "Young" Simpson.

At this point I began to look up the details of Simpson's election to the Chair. In spite of his youth — youth, that is, for an appointment of such high prestige at the age of twenty-nine — he presented an impressive, two hundred page volume of testimonials and references, together with a sixty page appendix in which his seven hundred museum specimens were catalogued. It is probable, therefore, that he felt that he was the best candidate by reason of his special knowledge and already extensive experience. Simpson was never lacking in self-confidence and had no false modesty. As for youth, he may well have considered that it was a sin which we all commit in our turn, or a bad habit which we all outgrow in later life.

He was unmarried when he applied for the appointment, and some of the electors expressed grave doubts as to whether an unmarried man could be considered for the particular work involved. At that time, the system of election was peculiar because Edinburgh's City Council took a prominent part in the selection of Professors; it may well have been that this objection concerning celibacy originated from one of the lay Councillors rather than from a medical source. Simpson dealt with this obstacle with his usual forthright and determined resolution. "Will you support my candidature if I get married before the day of the election?" He got married, the proprieties were satisfied and that obstruction was cleared out of the way.

The story about Simpson's name interested me, although it was of no real importance to anybody. Was it true, or not? Why had it hardly ever been mentioned in print? If it was true, what was the point of it? If it was not true, how had the tale originated?

I went, first, to my local library and consulted *Crockford's Clerical Directory* to obtain the name and address of the Anglican clergyman at Bathgate — Simpson's birthplace in West Lothian. Whether they were called "vicars" in Scotland I knew not, but the local incumbent, the Reverend Passmore, replied to my letter in some detail, even though he was unable to give any real help himself. Indirectly, however, he was of great assistance.

"I am afraid I can give you no direct help with your enquiry about Sir James Simpson.

"There was no Episcopal Church in Bathgate in 1811 and, in any case, I have always understood that he was a member of the Church of Scotland which, of course, is a Presbyterian Church.

"I have made enquiry of the Minister of the Bathgate Parish Church, and he tells me that all registers prior to 1850 have been sent to Edinburgh for safe keeping, so that he cannot even say with certainty if Simpson was baptised here. But if you will write to the Keeper of Documents, Tolbooth Church, Edinburgh, he will be able to refer to the Register . . . .

"I would only add that I think it highly unlikely that the 'Young' was a later addition: the use of the mother's maiden name, or of some other family name, as a middle name was already common at the beginning of the last century, and it was usually given at Baptism. Also, since I came to Bathgate, I have not heard any suggestion that he was ever known except as J.Y."

I took the Reverend Passmore's advice and wrote to the Tolbooth Church. The reply was headed "The Church of Scotland. General Assembly", so I seemed to be straying into high, ecclesiastical circles.

"The Records from the Tolbooth have now been lodged in the Register House, Edinburgh, and I think you should make application there . . . . Professor J. Y. Simpson was in the United Free Church before the Union of the Churches . . . and it is unlikely that his ancestors would be in the Episcopal Church . . . . The point you raise is an interesting one, although I have never heard it suggested . . . ."

I was, by now, getting somewhat confused about the various Churches in Scotland and so, as advised, I wrote to New Register House in Edinburgh and received a laconic, but conclusive, note from the Registrar General's Office for Scotland. It said:

"... the following entry relative to the birth of James Simpson has been traced in the Register of Births and Baptisms pertaining to the Parish of Bathgate, *viz*:—

> 1811, June 7th. David Simpson and his
> spouse Mary Tarvey had a child born.
> Bapt'd. the 30th. June James Simpson."

So, Simpson had not been given the name "Young" at his baptism and, presumably, had assumed it at some later date. Surprisingly, the rumour of which I had heard, turned out to be true, in spite of the absence of all written evidence in the literature; in spite of the fact that it was not generally known in Bathgate, his birthplace; in spite of the fact that an official of the General Assembly had never heard of it, and in spite of its improbability as pointed out by the Reverend Passmore. Nonetheless, there appears to be no loophole for error. There is no risk of confusion with another person — the date is correct, the place is correct and the parentage is correct.[2]

It may be that there is some prosaic explanation. It is possible that there was another James Simpson, perhaps in Bathgate, perhaps at the University, and that our James, mindful of the fact that, as far as he was concerned, only one James Simpson really mattered, made sure that there would be no confusion by taking an extra name. This would fit his character quite well; there was never any trace of an inferiority complex about the future discoverer of chloroform. The *Dictionary of National Biography* does list two other "James Simpsons" each of whom was a person of note, had strong connections with Edinburgh and, for some years (including the time of "our" James Simpson's appointment to his Chair of Midwifery), was contemporary with him.[2]

His adoption of his extra name may have been, as Dr. Armstrong Davison appeared to suggest, merely a symptom of his truculent and argumentative disposition. He may have thought, when he applied for the Professorship, "Is it a crime to be young? Must all Professors be past their best when appointed? I'll show them! I have the best credentials and experience, and, if these are ignored just because I am young, then I do not really want the job. I *am* young and not ashamed of it. What is more I will call myself 'Young' just to rub it in—they cannot then say that I am hiding anything." Of course, this is all conjectural, but it is entirely compatible with Simpson's forceful character. Whether it is correct or not is another matter: it is, at least, reasonable.

I am glad that I followed up this story and traced the entry in the Register of Births and Baptisms. Ever since I first heard of this rumour I was uneasily conscious that here was a loose end which should be tied up. A small point and an unimportant one, of no practical value at all, but worth tracking down as a matter of academic interest. Why the story never got into print until ninety years after his death I have no idea. Perhaps it was because having adopted the name he always used it; everything he wrote was signed "James Young Simpson" or "J. Y. Simpson". There is, however, no reason why the story should be witheld; it is unusual, very unusual, but not at all discreditable .

I was just about to close this essay with thanks to the people, mentioned above, who replied to my letter so helpfully and enabled me to solve the mystery when I realised, suddenly, that a loose end was still there. I had not, necessarily, reached the correct answer.

I said earlier that the date was correct, the place was correct and the parentage was correct, but this was not strictly accurate. The date and place I had, indeed, confirmed from my own card index, but for the parents' names I had relied on my memory. This is an appalling thing for a historian to have done—an unforgiveable sin. There are two essentials in history. The first is always to check your references and the second is to be no duller than necessary. To contravene the first law is to make one's efforts useless, unreliable and, possibly, misleading. To disobey the second law is merely to make history unreadable, which is not quite so serious. At least a dull history will not mislead its readers — it will have no readers!

When I realised my mistake in not having checked the names of Simpson's father and mother I proceeded to do so, with astonishing result. I began by looking at Sir James' obituaries in the two principal medical journals[3,4] and found that neither mentioned his parents by name at all. So, I turned once more to the *Dictionary of National Biography*[2] which stated that his father's name was David and he was the local baker in Bathgate. This agreed with the Registrar-General's letter. So far, so good. However the *Dictionary of National Biography* gave Sir James' mother's name as Mary Jervie, whereas the Registrar-General had said it was Mary Tarvey.

This discrepancy could have been due to a mis-reading of manuscript document compiled in the days before typewriters, but the matter could not be left there. Some degree of certainty had to be attained and this meant a further search. Therefore, I consulted Laing Gordon's book on Simpson and

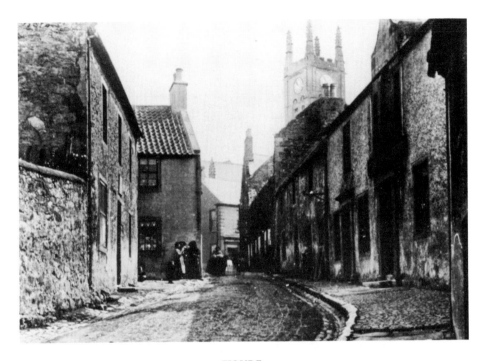

FIGURE 9
Sir James Simpson's birthplace in Bathgate, a town which lies between Edinburgh and Glasgow. The Simpsons' home was the house in the left foreground, and has now been demolished.

39

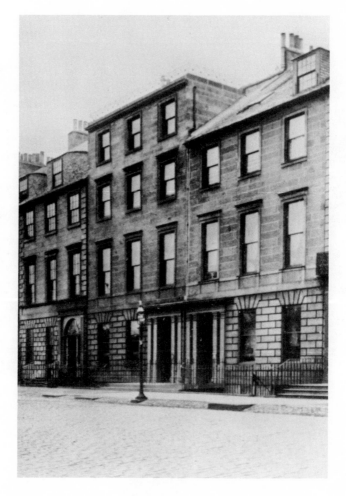

FIGURE 10
The house, at 52 Queen Street, Edinburgh, in which Simpson lived from 1845 until his death in 1870.

found that it gave an extract from the visiting book of the Bathgate doctor who attended Simpson's birth:[5]

"275. June 7. Simpson, David, baker, Bathgate. Wife Mary Jarvie Æ 40. 8th. child. son Natus 8 o'clock. Uti veniebam natus. Paid 10s. 6d."

This extract is also exactly reproduced as a footnote in Duns' *memoir of Sir James Y. Simpson*; in his text, however, the author says that the mother's name was "Jarvey".[6]

I next referred to Sir William Hale-White's book;[7] Sir William agreed with Laing Gordon, and the local doctor, and called her "Jarvie". Then, I consulted Eve Blantyre Simpson's life of Sir James.[8] Hers ought to be a reliable account for she was his daughter, and would, almost certainly, have known her grandmother's maiden name. Miss Simpson's account of her father's date and place of birth, and the name and occupation of her grandfather were as before — there was never any doubt about these — but her remarks on her grandmother's name were extremely interesting. It appeared that all the other variants were incorrect. Mrs. David Simpson was a descendant of a Huguenot family, which came to Britain from Guienne, named "Gervais", which name was later anglicised, or rather scotticised, into "Jervay". The name may, possibly, have been "Gervaise" (the only time Miss Simpson mentions it is in the plural form as "Gervaises"), but this seems much less likely. "Jervay" and "Gervais" fit much better phonetically.

We now have seven different forms of the name, derived from six different sources:

Registrar-General	Tarvey
Dictionary of National Biography	Jervie
Laing Gordon	Jarvie
Duns	Jarvie or Jarvey
Hale-White	Jarvie
Eve Simpson	Jervay (derived from Gervais, or Gervaise)

Eve Simpson's version, arguably, is the most reliable since she was writing about her own grandmother. The confusion which exists about the other variants has probably arisen from a variety of factors. Bad writing and spelling, less rigidly standardised than today, coupled with the different articulation of vowel sounds in Scotland, England and France seem to be the main ones.

The confusion and doubt about Mary Simpson's maiden name does not, however, alter my earlier conclusion that the future James Young Simpson assumed his middle name some time after his Baptism. The estimated population of Bathgate, in 1959, was 12,000 or so and there were quite a few families "Simpson" there. In 1811, however, Bathgate was just a village and, when I looked at the 1811 Census report, its population was recorded as being 2,919. The chances of another James Simpson being born on the same day of the same year to another David and Mary Simpson are, in a village of this size, infinitesimal, and so we can accept the Registrar-General's statement that our James was not given the name "Young" at his Baptism.

(When I was looking up the last fact in this tale of doubts and discrepancies — the population of Bathgate in 1811 — I found still one more inconsistency. The village according to my records, was in West Lothian. The Census figures for each town and village were given county by county and in alphabetical order; West Lothian, to my dismay, was not mentioned. I searched through the whole lot and, finally, found Bathgate's entry under the county of Linlithgow. Did this mean that there was more than just one village of this name? Apparently not, but why was West Lothian omitted? Was it a new county formed after 1811?

Most Scots will know the answer, but I had to turn to the *Encyclopaedia Britannica* for enlightenment; it explained that West Lothian and Linlithgow were alternative names for the same area.[9] (So it was the right village, after all!)

REFERENCES

[1] Armstrong Davison, M. H. (1960) The Evolution of Anaesthesia. *British Journal of Anaesthesia*, **32**, 141–146.

[2] Anonymous. (1909) Sir James Young Simpson. *Dictionary of National Biography*, London; Smith, Elder and Co.

[3] Anonymous. (1870) Obituary. Sir James Y. Simpson, Bart. *British Medical Journal*, **1**, 505–508.

[4] Anonymous. (1870) Obituary. Sir James Young Simpson. *Lancet*, **1**, 715–718.

[5] Gordon, H. L. (1897) *Sir James Young Simpson and Chloroform*, London: T. Fisher Unwin.

[6] Duns, J. (1893) *Memoir of Sir James Y. Simpson*, Edinburgh: Edmonston and Douglas.

[7] Hale-White, Sir W. (1935) *Great Doctors of the Nineteenth Century*, London: Arnold.

[8] Simpson, E. B. (1896) *Sir James Y. Simpson*, Edinburgh: Oliphant, Anderson and Ferrier.

[9] Anonymous. (1946) Linlithgow. In *Encyclopaedia Britannica*, Chicago: Encyclopaedia Britannica Inc.

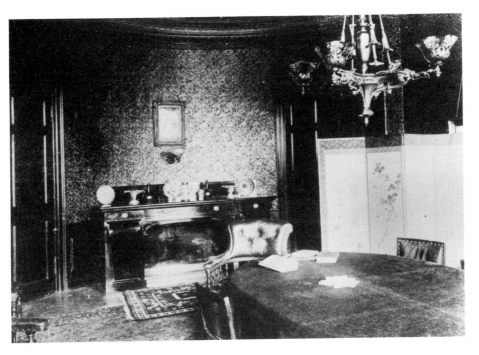

FIGURE 11

The dining room of Simpson's home in Edinburgh. Here, on the 4th November, 1847 Simpson himself, Matthews Duncan, George Keith and Miss Petrie (Simpson's niece) chloroformed themselves around the dining table. Mrs. Petrie later became Mrs. Agnes Thompson; she lived until January 1914.

CHAPTER 5

THE JUMP-UP-BEHINDER

One week after the first news of anaesthesia broke upon the United Kingdom, in 1847,[1] there was a letter to the Editor of *The Lancet* from Dr. Robert H. Collyer whose address, then, was in St. Helier, the capital of the Channel Island of Jersey.

"I have seen, by the communication in *The Lancet* of last week, that Mr. Liston has lately performed an operation on a person rendered unconscious by the inhalation of narcotic and stimulating vapours. The credit of the discovery is given to Dr. Morton, of Boston, U.S.

"In the early part of the year 1843, I published a work in Boston, U.S., wherein, at page twenty-six, I distinctly declare, that '*a congestive* or unconscious state may be induced by the inhalation of narcotic or stimulating vapours.' I made the experiment on about twenty persons, and found that the condition so induced was difficult to manage.

"I am sure you will give this insertion, in order that, if the application of stimulating vapours through the respiratory organs should be found productive of the greatest of human blessings, the alleviation of pain, I may at least enjoy the credit of having first suggested the idea to the world."[2]

Four weeks later, Dr. Collyer again wrote to *The Lancet*. This time, he wrote of Morton's attempt to patent for himself the invention of ether (which he called "Letheon"); Collyer regarded this with righteous indignation.

"The idea of trading, bartering, and speculating, on the 'ills that flesh is heir to', is to me a most revolting thought; it bespeaks a condition of mind unworthy of our noble profession.

"Years since, I gave the process of inhalation to produce unconsciousness to the world, without the most remote idea of remuneration, which I thought was amply afforded me in the knowledge that I had contributed towards the alleviating of suffering humanity. The process of inhalation to produce unconsciousness, so that all kinds of surgical operations might be performed without pain to the patient, I have publicly advocated since 1842 and published in 1843. I am not responsible for the apathy manifested from that time to the present moment, when it seems to have flashed on the profession as if by magic, and is now generally adopted.

"I now distinctly give to all who may choose to use it, 'the process of inhalation for the production of unconsciousness, so that surgical operations can be performed without pain to the patient'. I do this without fear or compromise, knowing that I can substantiate my claim to priority. And if any patent is taken out, I will take measures to render it null and void."[3]

The Editor of *The Lancet*, on publishing this far-reaching claim, showed a cautious reserve, and added a comment of his own.

"Dr. Collyer should produce something like proof of his liberality. In the first instance, proof should be given that the discovery of the production of insensibility by ether, and its application to surgery, were his to give. As yet, nothing of this kind has been supplied, and until it is, the writer must be content to belong to the class of jump-up-behinders."

This cold douche of acid comment was typical of Mr. Thomas Wakley who was, at the time, the Editor of *The Lancet*. In the event, it failed to produce a reply from Dr. Collyer — I could find no further letters from him or about him, for at least 21 years. Then, in 1868, a letter was published above the simple pen-name of "Anaesthesia"; I do not think there can be much doubt, after reading the letter, that the author was Dr. Collyer.

"The following is the chronological history of painless surgical operations during the anaesthetic state, induced by the inhalation of narcotic and stimulating vapours:—
"The first surgical operation during an anaesthetic condition, induced by the inhalation of the fumes from rum, was the reduction of a dislocation of the hip-joint of a negro, 'Bob'. Louisiana. By Dr. Collyer. December, 1839.
"Extraction of tooth from Miss Mary Allen during an insensible condition, induced by the inhalation of ether combined with the fumes from poppy-seeds. Philadelphia. By Dr. Collyer. November, 1842.
"Publication of 'Psychography' (copyrighted work), wherein at pages 26, 27, and 28, particular mention is made that the inhalation of narcotic and stimulating vapours will produce the anaesthetic state. Philadelphia. By Dr. Collyer. May, 1843.
"Insensibility produced by the inhalation of protoxide of nitrogen. Hartford, Connecticut. Horace Wells, 1845.
"Publication in *Boston Medical Journal*, that ether combined with opium would produce the anaesthetic state. Boston. By Dr. Smilie. June, 1846.
"Administration of ether by Drs. Morton and Jackson. Boston, United States. September, 1846.
"Inhalation of chloroform. Edinburgh. By Dr. Simpson, 1854.
"Amylene, London. By Dr. Snow. 1857.
"Bichloride of methylene. London. By Dr. Richardson. 1867."[4]

There are a number of inaccuracies in this letter. Two years later, in 1870, there was one more reference to Dr. Collyer in the pages of *The Lancet*.

"Amongst the pioneers in the practice of inhalation was an enthusiast whose name has never yet been recognised by the profession, but whose services ought certainly not to be overlooked. We refer to Dr. Robert H. Collyer. Dr. Collyer was a pupil of Dr. Turner, the Professor of Chemistry of University College; he was an active student of chemistry, and at the same time an ardent believer in mesmerism. In 1835 Collyer was present at Professor Turner's lecture when some experiments on the inhalation of ether were performed; he himself was made insensible with ether, and observed that his fellow-students who inhaled it were insensible to pain. In 1839 he had returned to America, where his father resided near to New Orleans, and in December of that year he was called to one of the negroes on his father's establishment who had been rendered insensible by inhaling the fumes from a vat of rum, and who on falling had dislocated his hip. Finding the muscles flaccid, Dr. Collyer reduced the dislocation without exciting the least sensation of pain in the patient. Afterwards he began to practise mesmeric procedures, and in two cases of surgical operation he seems to have been successful. These facts led him to connect the phenomena of mesmerism with those of narcotism produced by inhaling narcotic vapours; and in the years immediately succeeding 1839 he lectured in America, before large audiences, on these subjects. In 1843 he came to Liverpool and we have before us a copy of the *Liverpool Mail* of Oct. 14th of the year named (1843), which contains nearly a column of abstract of one of his lectures. In the same year he published a book called 'Psychography', bearing on his favourite themes. The lectures and works of Dr. Collyer were of a kind, we must candidly say, not calculated to arrest seriously the attention of the profession at that time; and his experiments, in some of which he resorted to mesmerism, and in others to the administration of the fumes of alcohol in which poppy-seeds and coriander had been steeped, were popular rather than scientific in their nature. But there is this principle pervading them all — a principle he incessantly promulgated in Boston, Philadelphia, Liverpool, and other places — that the so-called mesmeric influence was identical in action with that induced by inhaling narcotic and stimulating vapours. He theorised, moreover, on the conditions of brain in those susceptible to its influence; that during the congestive state the brain did not receive impressions from the rest of the body, but was, so to speak, cut off from connexion with the body for the time; and that under the influence of narcotic vapours the same congestive condition of the brain obtained In 1842 he claims to have administered the fumes of his alcoholic mixture to a Mrs. Allen, of Philadelphia, while a tooth was extracted, without pain.

"It is difficult to estimate what effect Dr. Collyer's lectures and writings had upon the direct progress of discovery; but as, at the time we name, they excited great general attention, as the lectures were delivered in various places and before large audiences and were commented on freely by the public press, and as his writings were disseminated broadcast, it is next to impossible to assume that they did not direct the minds of men to the subject of inhalation for the purpose of producing temporary insensibility to pain. Anyway, it is one of the strangest of coincidences, if it be a coincidence, that the development of the anaesthetic process took place immediately after Collyer's public exhibitions, and in the very centres where his lectures had been delivered.

"From the time when the process of anaesthesia by inhalation was established to the present time Dr. Collyer (for he is still alive) has persistently maintained his priority of claim as the suggestor of the practice, while he has assigned, as is correct, to Sir Humphry Davy, the origination of the principle. How far his claim is sustainable, our readers, with the simple facts now before them, can judge independently. Our own opinion is that Collyer, a man of impetuous perception, impulsive action, open nature, and unrestrainable fluency of speech, did originally seize such analogies as exist between the so-called hypnotic condition from mesmerism and the rapid narcotism produced by narcotic vapours; that he laid himself out publicly to announce these analogies; that he succeeded in securing a violent opposition, which made his peculiar views familiar to those who were living near the scene of controversy; and that he cried first hail on a beat which he did not follow up efficiently. We have, further, no doubt that had he given up the mesmeric idea and proceeded systematically with his plan of making the body insensible by inhaling the vapour of alcohol, he would have had no-one to dispute with him in priority. As it was, after throwing out a fine suggestion, he virtually deserted it himself, as if he did not himself see the whole of its extensive application and importance. In this respect Dr. Collyer simply represents a constantly repeated figure in the history of human effort. He is Prince Rupert to the life, not to mention other men of similar impulsive genius in other ages and on different fields of labour. . . .

"Let us close the controversy. Enthusiast Collyer, wandering through the States with his mesmerism and narcotic fumes; his ancedotes of the Pythoness of the Delphic oracle who inhaled such fumes, of the Egyptian magi, of his negro 'Bob' undergoing operation insensible from the inhalation of rum, of himself insensible from inhalation of ether in the laboratory of University College, and with his theories of mesmeric sleep in connexion with sleep from narcotic and stimulating vapours, and hybernation — enthusiast Collyer, we say, is to our minds the true modern pioneer after all — the man who ran first, and beckoned and called, however oddly, others to follow, with so much effect that a few followed at once, and many afterwards."[5]

What are we to make of the above strange mixture? *The Lancet* at first, and very rightly, asked for evidence of Collyer's claim — evidence which was never supplied. Later, the same journal veered round and, without mentioning its earlier disparagement of Collyer, accorded him a great deal of credit in the discovery of anaesthesia. I was surprised at this inconsistency and unable to explain it. When, however, I gave the first draft of this essay to Nan, my wife, to read she asked at once "Had old Mr. Wakely retired by this time?"

That, of course, was it. Mr. Thomas Wakely had not only retired, but had died, and he, with his stormy and pugnacious personality, had been replaced by his two sons who were softer, less forthright, more polite and more credulous than their caustic-tongued father.

It was very evident that I had to read Dr. Collyer's own book and discover what evidence it contained, for it was upon this publication that he based his claim. Collyer did not give its title in his signed letters, but his *alter ego* "Anaesthesia" did, as did *The Lancet* in 1870. Collyer's book has the usual, snappy, nineteenth century title of twenty-five words, in almost as many different kinds of type. *Psychography, or, the Embodiment of Thought; with an analysis of phreno-magnetism, "neurology", and mental hallucination, including rules to govern and produce the magnetic state.*[6] It is, in other words, a book on hypnotism, with curious theories and statements which are obscure and difficult to understand. In it mesmerism, animal magnetism, and clairvoyance are all mixed up with phrenology and psychography whereas phreno-magnetism and "neurology" (whatever they were) are not at all the same and should not be confused with true magnetism or the congestive state. Collyer alluded to the phenomenon of persistence of vision, and compared it with the experiments of Daguerre who first produced permanent pictures on iodised silver plates (daguerrotypes) in 1839.

Nowhere in his book did Collyer ever mention using ether, or using mesmerism to relieve pain or to produce anaesthesia during surgery. It is quite clear that Collyer's thoughts, when he wrote his treatise, were not running in the direction of painless surgery at all. In his first letter to *The Lancet* he referred to page twenty-six of his book "wherein, . . . I distinctly declare that '*a congestive* or unconscious state may be induced by the inhalation of narcotic or stimulating vapours'." The following quotation is taken from that page, and is the only reference in the book which, in any way, bears on the point in question.

"The magnetic or congestive state of the brain is often accompanied by that exalted condition of mind, called clairvoyance. Then, the faculties seem to have hardly a limit of action; time and space are annihilated; the secrets of the past, present and future are brought within the immediate range of thought.

"The power to induce this state of the nervous system is not confined to the nervo-vital fluid, from a second person. The same state of things may be brought about by mental excitement, accompanied with muscular action; the inhaling of narcotic and stimulating vapors; the abnormal condition, as manifested in Somnambulism, Trance, Catalepsy, or by the will of the individual himself, as was the case with Apollonius of Tyana, Emanuel Swedenborg, Mahomet, &c."

Who knows what Collyer may have had in mind when he wrote his

49

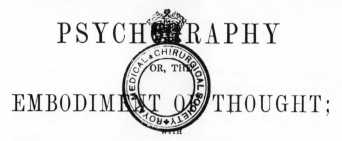

PSYCHOGRAPHY

OR, THE

EMBODIMENT OF THOUGHT;

AN ANALYSIS OF PHRENO-MAGNETISM, "NEUROLOGY,"
AND MENTAL HALLUCINATION,

INCLUDING

RULES TO GOVERN AND PRODUCE THE MAGNETIC STATE.

———————

EXPERIMENT WITH THE "BOWL OF MOLASSES."

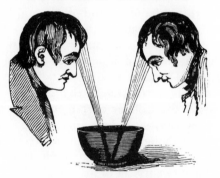

Let them laugh at me for speaking of things which they do not understand; and I must pity them while they laugh at me.—*St. Austin.*

———————

BY ROBT. H. COLLYER, M.D.

MEMBER OF MASSACHUSETTS MEDICAL SOCIETY, (LATE PUPIL OF DR. ELLIOTSON, AT THE LONDON UNIVERSITY,) &c. &c.

—————

SOLD BY ZIEBER & CO., PHILADELPHIA; SUN OFFICE, NEW YORK; REDDING & CO., BOSTON.

....

1843.

FIGURE 12
The title page of Collyer's book *Psychography* in which, it was mistakenly claimed, the first suggestion of ether anaesthesia was made.

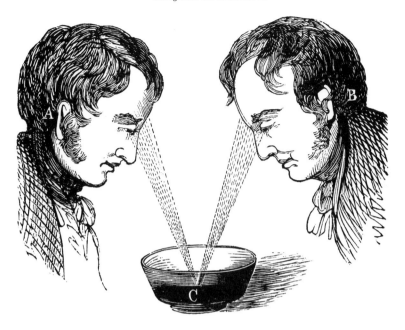

FIGURE 13

It is quite clear that Collyer's thoughts were not running in the direction of painless surgery at all. He believed that the "resident principle of the brain" was subject to the same physical laws as heat, light and electricity. "The knowledge of this law prepared me for the experiment of *reflecting thoughts* in a proper medium. When I announced, in January last, my performance with the 'cup of molasses', I was not surprised at the ridicule it met with from the editors throughout the land."

book? But he certainly did not write of an unconscious state — merely of a magnetic or congestive state of the brain. On pages twenty-seven and twenty-eight of the book (which were cited as supporting evidence for Collyer's claim by the anonymous "Anaesthesia" in 1868) there are accounts of the Delphic oracle and of the antics of a man in Cairo who demonstrated thought-reading.

"The particular apartment of the oracle was immediately over the chasm from which the vapors issued. A priestess delivered the responses. . . . She sat upon a tripod or three-legged stool, perforated with holes, over the seat of the vapors. After a time, her figure enlarged itself, her hair stood on end, her complexion and features became altered, her heart panted, her bosom swelled, and her voice grew more than human. In this condition, she uttered words which were supposed to be dictated by the god. . . . The condition of the priestess was identical with that of a mesmerized person. . . . .

51

"Lord Prudhoe and Major Felix being at Cairo last autumn . . . found the town in a state of extraordinary excitement, in consequence of the recent arrival in those parts of a celebrated magician . . . [who] . . . exercised the power of showing to any visiter [sic] who chose to comply with his terms, any persons, dead or living, whom the same visiter pleased to name. . . . A pure seer, to wit, a maiden's eye, or a boy was required; these are constitutionally more susceptible to the influence of the narcotic fumes. I find that, with very little trouble, they are easily subdued by the nervous agency; whereas strong persons, as men and older women, are very hard to be affected. . . ."

The magician "kindled some spices on a sort of small altar in the middle of the room . . . and poured about a table-spoonful of some black liquid into the boy's right hand and bade him hold the hand steady, and keep his eye fixed upon the surface of the liquid . . . the angle of direction from the boy's mind must be in accordance with the angle from the person in correspondence". Then members of the audience were invited to name any person they wished to the magician — Shakespeare, Voltaire, the brother of Major Felix, and others. The boy, seemingly under the influence of the fumes, and peering, as directed, at the "reflection" from the black liquid in his palm, described each one in turn. "The major swooned away."

Well, that particular member of the British Army may have been impressed, but neither of these descriptions applies at all to inhalational anaesthesia. The substances inhaled are not mentioned or described, those who inhaled were not unconscious — quite the contrary, they spoke throughout the procedure — there is no reference whatsoever to ether, and the purpose for which the inhalations took place was not for the relief of pain. Out of his own mouth, therefore, Dr. Collyer's bombastic and impudent claim to be the originator of anaesthesia is revealed to be without any real foundation.

Collyer appears, from his writings, to have been eccentric and unconventional. No harm in that at all. The obscure subjects about which he wrote were, and still are, well worth investigating. But the claim he founded on a few casual sentences unrelated to its subject was so far divorced from reality that it passes the bounds of normal. He was either an unscrupulous crook and twister or, in one respect at least, he was not quite sane. He resembled Charles T. Jackson in his anxiety to claim credit for a discovery made by others. Jackson died insane — I wonder if the same thing happened to Collyer?

He was certainly a man with a grievance. In a preface to *Psychography* written to Dr. Winslow Lewis, of Boston, he said:

"When a malicious and unprincipled herd would have crushed me you came to my rescue. You knew me to be engaged in the advocacy of a solemn truth, one which must revolutionise the false philosophy of past ages; one which opens to man the secret of his immortality; . . . one which, in a medical point of view, will tend more to alleviate suffering humanity, than all the multitude of medicaments, from the time of Galen to the present day. It is scarce three years since I publicly espoused the cause, I was heralded with scoffs, jeers, licentious ribaldry, ridicule, and all the artillery which puny scribblers could bring to bear."

And, he had no small opinion of his own work.

"The Brain is the most delicate instrument within the whole range of nature; its office is one which brings man in contact with the world; it is the medium of his external consciousness, and is the residence of that imperishable soul, which is as eternal as God Himself. The phenomena of its operations are so eminently above all other conditions of matter, that it paralyzes the mightiest minds in the investigation. . . . I have, after years of untiring exertion, arrived at conclusions which are perfectly compatible with the experience of past ages. . . . I know that my age will not give me the credit I demand, but I know that posterity will carry out what I have begun, . . . then will these experiments take their proper rank in the temple of knowledge; . . . they will form the cupola of human attainment."

It is worth noting that Collyer's claims increased with the passage of time. His first letter merely claimed that a "congestive or unconscious state may be produced by the inhalation of narcotic and stimulating vapours". (There was no reference to unconsciousness in his book.) His second letter put the date one year earlier, and claimed that he had publicly advocated unconsciousness for operations since this time. In his book, surgical operations were never even mentioned. In the third letter, signed "Anaesthesia", two operations under anaesthesia by Dr. Collyer are mentioned, at very early dates — December, 1839 and November, 1842. Since this letter was anonymous, it may be said that it is not evidence either for or against him. I think it is almost certain, however, that he wrote it himself. The phrases are his, and it claims for him the first three places in the chronology of anaesthesia, antedating Horace Wells by two years and more.

Whoever wrote the letter their chronology is not very trustworthy. Of the last four items, three are wrong. Amylene was not first used in 1857; Snow, himself, stated that he first used it in 1856.[7] Simpson, of course, did not discover chloroform in 1854, but in 1847. The statement that Morton and Jackson used ether in September, 1846 is erroneous; Morton did, in the case of Eben Frost, but Jackson never saw an anaesthetic given until much later. The other inaccuracy is the statement that Collyer's book *Psychography* says that vapours will produce the anaesthetic state: it said nothing of the sort. Here, then, in a chronology consisting of nine items are four mistakes. I hope I will be forgiven for not attaching much importance to the other five items.

I entirely agree with Mr. Thomas Wakely's description of Dr. Robert H. Collyer as a jump-up-behinder.

*　　　*　　　*　　　*

Months after this essay was completed I came across another book written by Robert H. Collyer. It was published long after *Psychography*, not until 1871 in fact, which goes far to support my contention that Dr. Collyer could well have written the letter signed "Anaesthesia" in 1868.

This book, like his former one, is a curious mixture of subjects on the borderline between physiology, psychology and quackery. It has a grandiose title. *Mysteries of the vital element in connexion with dreams, somnambulism, trance, vital photography, faith and will, anaesthesia, nervous congestion and causative function. Modern Spiritualism explained.*[8]

Collyer devoted much of the first part of this book to anaesthesia, a subject on which we know he held very strong views. He stated that the first authentically recorded surgical operation without pain was performed in April, 1829 by Jules Cloquet who removed a breast for carcinoma under mesmerism or "a nervous congestive state of the brain". Collyer claimed to have repeated this, in 1841, in a child aged 22 months, for extirpation of an eye. He reiterated his experiences with "Bob" and of inhalation of ether at University College in London and went on:

"For nearly a quarter of a century I have been defrauded of my just rights as the original discoverer; every species of misrepresentation and special pleading has been resorted to to deceive and mislead the public".

Collyer gave fuller descriptions of his own, early cases. The child's eye was excised for a new growth in 35 minutes after he had mesmerised the patient. Two years earlier, in December, 1839, his father had heard laughter one Sunday afternoon, when there should have been no laughter. This happened at a plantation and distillery which produced up to 3,000 gallons of rum each day. On investigation, his father had found that some of the negro slaves had got into the distillery through the cellar; one of them, called Bob, had inhaled the fumes and fallen ten feet from the top of the vat. Collyer, having found that Bob's hip was dislocated, reduced it during the patient's unconsciousness. He then quoted the popular press (*The Boston Daily Ledger* of May 28th, 1842) to the effect that he had extracted teeth without pain in a mesmerised patient. Collyer claimed that W.T.G. Morton had been present, and saw this done. He gave the correct date of the arrival of the Cunarder *Acadia* bringing the news of anaesthesia to England. This tallies with the information I discovered, and which I have not seen published in earlier histories of anaesthesia. He then printed a certificate, dated January 2nd, 1847, stating that during one of his lectures on the tenth of December, 1846 in St. Helier, Jersey, the eighteen signatories

"Were present at a lecture delivered by Dr. Collyer ... in this town. We distinctly heard him state, that he had frequently, by the inhalation of narcotic and stimulant vapours, brought about a state of unconsciousness like that produced by the mesmeric passages, and that during that state all kinds of surgical operations could be performed without pain to the patient."

This was nearly a week before the arrival, in Liverpool, of the *Acadia*. Collyer then argued that this was exactly what he had claimed in his earlier book on *Psychography*. This was quite incorrect, and is the weak point of his whole case. He admitted that honour was due to Morton, rather than Jackson, but added that neither Morton, Wells nor Jackson made any other original discoveries. He listed his own as follows:

1842	Improved method of making sugar.
1851	New method of crushing quartz.
1852	New amalgamating apparatus.
1854	Improved breech-loading cannon.
1859	New coating for iron ships.
1860	New paper materials. (also 1861)
1862	New machine for cleaning grain.
1862	Chemical ink-pencil.
1862	New insulating covering for telegraph cables.
1863	New chemical tubing.
1870	Machine for treating flax.

In addition to these material things, he claimed the discovery of induced mental hallucination or electro-biology, of phreno-magnetism and vital photography. Each of these, however true, is completely irrelevant to Collyer's claim to be the discoverer of modern anaesthesia. Thereafter, the book wanders off into a number of by-paths — animal magnetism, mesmerism or nervous congestion, clairvoyance, Egyptian mysteries, somnambulism, necromancy, dreams, hallucinations, vital photography, creative function, faith and will, morale, spiritualism, and will power as anti-gravity. Electric eels, surprisingly (perhaps not surprisingly) make their appearance in this strange work. I fear that my own mind is not agile enough, nor sufficiently protean, to follow Dr. Collyer into all these side-tracks, and to weave them into one coherent whole.

He then gave a longer, and more detailed chronology of anaesthesia, in which three places were reserved for himself. This version was much more accurate, as far as dates are concerned, than that which appeared in the earlier letter by "Anaesthesia". It seems that, by this time, Dr. Collyer had checked his references much more carefully.

Nowhere, after his initial letter to *The Lancet*, does Collyer mention his experiment with inhalation of narcotic vapours "on about twenty persons". He may have reduced Bob's dislocated hip during anaesthesia produced by rum; he may have been successful in using mesmerism for operations, but neither of these things was particularly original. Both had been done before. That is the most that I am inclined to allow him.

This second book of Collyer's produces no fresh evidence that he was the originator of inhalational anaesthesia. His claim for this still rests solely upon his statement in *Psychography*, and close examination of both books reveals that the claim he made was irrelevant.

Dr. Collyer failed to make out his case — either at the time, or viewed, later, with the perspective of history.

REFERENCES

[1] Boott, F. (1847) Surgical operations performed during insensibility. *Lancet*, **1**, 5–8.
[2] Collyer, R.H. (1847) Inhalation of narcotic vapour. *Lancet*, **1**, 50–51.
[3] Collyer, R.H. (1847) Patent for inhalation! *Lancet*, **1**, 163.
[4] "Anaesthesia" (1868) Operations under anaesthesia. *Lancet*, **1**, 112.
[5] Anonymous (1870) The History of Anaesthetic Discovery II. *Lancet*, **1**, 840–844.
[6] Collyer, R.H. (1843) *Psychography, or, the embodiment of thought; an analysis of phreno-magnetism 'neurology', and mental hallucination, including rules to govern and produce the magnetic state.* Philadelphia: Zieber.
[7] Anonymous (1857) On the vapour of amylene. *Lancet*, **1**, 63–64.
[8] Collyer, R.H. (1871) *Mysteries of the vital element in connexion with dreams, somnambulism, trance, vital photography, faith and will, anaesthesia, nervous congestion and causative function. Modern spiritualism explained.* London: Renshaw.

An editorial footnote :—

Yet another book on the subject was written by Dr. Collyer, and was published in 1877. It deals specifically with anaesthesia (as Collyer saw it) and its title is *Early History of the Anaesthetic Discovery; or painless surgical operations*.[1] The author's full name, Robert Hanham Collyer appears above

EARLY HISTORY

OF THE

ANÆSTHETIC DISCOVERY;

OR

PAINLESS SURGICAL OPERATIONS.

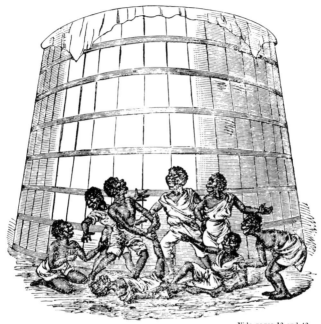

Vide pages 12 and 13.

In a paper read before the British Association, 1869, by Benjamin W. Richardson, M.D., F.R.S,, he says—"The ALCOHOLS are strictly anæsthetics, and indeed the first published case of a surgical operation under anæsthetic sleep by inhalation was performed by Dr. COLLYER, on a person rendered insensible by breathing the fumes of alcohol."

By ROBERT HANHAM COLLYER, M.D.,

ORIGINAL DISCOVERER OF THE NITROUS-OXIDE, ETHER, AND CHLOROFORM PROCESS

LONDON:
H. VICKERS, 317, STRAND.

1877.

Price 2*s.* 6*d.*

FIGURE 14

The title page of Collyer's *Early History of the Anaesthetic discovery* which shows what happened to Bob and his friends when they inhaled from the vat of rum.

57

the legend "Original discoverer of the nitrous oxide, ether and chloroform process". The title page also has an illustration showing what happened when Bob and his friends inhaled the vapour from the vat of rum.

Early on in his introduction, Collyer wrote.

"I inherited a more than usual sensitively sympathetic disposition, more especially for the sufferings and pains of others, and shunned the society of those who indulged in cruelty to lower animals. It is somewhat strange that being so constituted I should have chosen medicine and surgery as my profession."

He acknowledged the importance of Humphry Davy's suggestion concerning the breathing of nitrous oxide during surgical operations and was able to recall the time when, as a schoolboy of seven years old, he had met that great man; that meeting had, he wrote, a lasting effect upon him. Collyer then reviewed his early experiences and repeated his claim, based on the passage which appeared on page twenty-six of *Psychography*. On this occasion he added an important word in brackets which most certainly did not appear in the original version.

"My language is not ambiguous, but is expressed in words which cannot admit of two interpretations — I there say, 'The nervous congestive state (Anaesthetic) can be produced by the inhalation of narcotic and stimulating vapours'."

Collyer justified this inclusion by saying that whenever he had written of "nervous congestion" he had implied, or stated, and always certainly meant that this term should be synonymous with the unconsciousness produced by anaesthesia (and by fainting, incidentally).

The peripatetic Dr. Collyer visited many parts of the world, going from London to France and America, where, in 1839 he completed his medical education which had been cut short in England for "unforseen family reasons". Thereafter, he travelled extensively over the North American continent and revisited the United Kingdom. During these wanderings, unfortunately, Dr. Collyer lost most of his original documents which, he assured his readers, would have proved his claim beyond doubt. (Most were destroyed during fires in San Francisco and London; others were stolen by Mexican bandits.)

The fifth reference quoted by Dr. Sykes, the anonymous "History of Anaesthetic Discovery" was the second part of three articles published by *The Lancet* on the occasion of the death of Sir James Simpson.[2,3,4] It is clear from Collyer's 1877 book that the author of these articles was Benjamin Ward Richardson. He had been lavish with his praise of Collyer and, for reasons which can no longer be fathomed, awarded him far more credit for the discovery of anaesthesia than was his due. Dr. Collyer, however, was not at all pleased, and took the view that Richardson had, in actual fact, belittled and derided him. He considered that Richardson had made a most important mistake by confusing the term "congestion of the brain" with that of "nervous congestion of the brain". To Collyer, the first meant an increased blood flow to the brain, and the second meant anaesthesia. An acrimonious exchange of correspondence between the two men ensued and eventually Richardson brought it to a close.

"Since receiving your last, I have recast all that I have written on the history of Anaesthesia, and my sincere and unchanged conviction is, that to add anything would be to spoil all that I have done. I should accept it as one of the worst things to be moved from the present good position in which you now stand; you must permit me to say, that I cannot write a word further for publication than I have written."

None of this correspondence was published in *The Lancet* and Collyer made a great deal of it in this book.

"Dr. Richardson, having put me in the wrong on a most important question, whether by misadventure or otherwise it matters not, it was his bounden duty, the moment his attention was called to the fact, to have corrected the error. . . .

"Having fought single-handed the great battle of Anaesthesia for nearly six years against all the prejudices, bigotry, superstition and ignorance of the age, receiving nothing but abuse and ridicule as my reward, it is not asking too much, now that the victory has been so signally achieved by the adoption of Anaesthetics in surgical operations, that I should have the full and entire credit which to myself belongs, namely, that of having caused the subject to be brought prominently before the public, and ultimately, as a consequence, the alleviation of human suffering, and the entire abolition of pain during surgical operations. . . . The mere substitution of one substance for another in the production of the Anaesthetic state, after the GREAT PRINCIPLE had been published by me in May, 1843, does not constitute DISCOVERY, nor does it demand any amount of research. . . .

"I am now, after seven years, convinced that Dr. Richardson was not competent to have written 'the History of Anaesthesia' from a want of knowledge of the facts, as they occurred in 1842 and 1843."

By this time Dr. Richardson must have regretted whatever it was that made him write such a fulsome account of Collyer and his work seven years previously.

The rest of Dr. Collyer's book consists of ever more detailed accounts of his own views and actions, and of the persecution meted out to him by others, together with long arguments which attempt to deny the work of those amongst whom varying degrees of priority had been distributed. No new evidence to support his original claim is to be found in the 72 pages of this book. Having read it, however, one can appreciate why Dr. Sykes, in his essay, thought fit to question Collyer's sanity. Neither Dr. Sykes then, nor I now, are competent to pronounce on this subject.

To sum up any dispute concerning to whom should priority be accorded for the introduction of anaesthesia there are no better words than those used, in 1917, by Sir William Osler.

"Time out of mind, patients have been rendered insensible by potions or vapors, or by other methods, without any one man forcing any one method into general acceptance, or influencing in any way surgical practice.

"Before October 16, 1846, surgical anaesthesia did not exist — within a few months it became a world-wide procedure; and the full credit for its introduction must be given to William Thomas Green Morton, who, on the date mentioned, demonstrated at the Massachusetts General Hospital the simplicity and safety of ether anaesthesia. On the priority question let me quote two appropriate paragraphs — He becomes the true discoverer who establishes the truth; and the sign of the truth is the general acceptance. Whoever, therefore, resumes the investigation of neglected or repudiated doctrine, elicits its true demonstration, and discovers and explains the nature of the errors which have led to its tacit or declared rejection, may certainly and confidently await the acknowledgment of his right in its discovery. In science the credit goes to the man who convinces the world, not to the man to whom the idea first occurs. Morton convinced the world: the credit is his."[5]

REFERENCES

[1] Collyer, R.H. (1877) *Early History of the Anaesthetic Discovery; or painless surgical operations. With letters to and from Sir James Y. Simpson, Dr. Benjamin W. Richardson, and Dr. Henry Bennet. Boston versus Hartford.* London: Vickers.

[2] Anonymous (1870) The History of Anaesthetic Discovery. *Lancet*, 1, 770–772.

[3] Anonymous (1870) The History of Anaesthetic Discovery. *Lancet*, 1, 840–844.

[4] Anonymous (1870) The History of Anaesthetic Discovery. *Lancet*, 2, 16–18.

[5] Osler, W. (1917) The first printed documents relating to modern surgical anaesthesia. *Annals of Medical History*, 1, 329–332.

CHAPTER 6

DEPHLOGISTICATED AIR

Joseph Priestley was born on the 13th November, 1733 at Fieldhead, Birstall, Yorkshire. The house in which he was born was demolished in 1858, but its successor has a plaque to mark the site and commemorate the event.

Priestley was ordained as a Nonconformist Minister in 1762 and, thereafter, led an unsettled and occasionally stormy life. He taught himself many oriental languages for the purpose of Bible study, and his literary output was varied and immense. The mere list of his writings in the *Dictionary of National Biography* occupies seven and a half columns, and is classified under the headings of theology, philology, history, politics, psychology and metaphysics, and science.

He was a Minister in many different places, in some of which he also acted as schoolmaster. His religious ideas went through a process of development and change and this may have accounted for his frequent removals. When, in 1767, he was at the Mill Hill Chapel in Leeds he studied "airs" which was the name by which gases were then known. His house was next door to a brewery and so he was able to obtain virtually unlimited quantities of "fixed air" (carbon dioxide) from the vats. He found, amongst other facts, that this gas dissolved in water when under pressure and thus, casually, invented soda water. He had had no formal training as a chemist, and was further handicapped by the complicated and preposterous Phlogiston Theory which made what was a difficult study almost impossible. Priestley was elected a Fellow of The Royal Society in 1766.

He ascertained that plants absorbed carbon dioxide, and gave out oxygen — which he called "dephlogisticated air". He devised the pneumatic trough as a convenient way of collecting gases for study, and introduced mercury as its liquid when dealing with gases which were soluble in water.

In 1791, when he was living in Birmingham, a Reform Society gave a dinner to celebrate the anniversary of the fall of the Bastille. The Society was far from revolutionary, its main activities being directed towards the abolition of the Slave Trade and the iniquitous Test Acts. Although Priestley had little connection with it he was thought to be sympathetic to the French Revolution and, as a result, his home was attacked by a mob. Most of his books, papers and instruments were destroyed. Two years later he emigrated to North America, and settled in Pennsylvania. He lived there, without becoming a naturalised American citizen, until his death on the 6th February, 1804.

Priestley's work *Experiments and Observations on Different Kinds of Air* was published in 1775,[1] and, on reading it, one can realise that the author had his feet planted very firmly on the ground right from the beginning; for he said:

"Prejudices . . . unknown to ourselves, bias not only our judgements, properly so called, but even the perceptions of our senses: for we may take a maxim so strongly for granted, that the plainest evidence of sense will not entirely change, and often hardly modify our persuasions . . ."

How right he was. No better example could be found than Edward Lawrie — of whom more later, in another essay — whose fixed idea that chloroform was perfectly harmless could not be altered or weakened by any number of deaths and disasters. Nothing could alter his preconceived opinions. Priestley, however, successfully overcame his ingrained beliefs and prejudices when he realised that the facts led him in a different direction.

"There are, I believe, very few maxims in philosophy that have laid firmer hold upon the mind, than that air, meaning atmospherical air . . . is a simple elementary substance, indestructible and unalterable. I was, however, soon satisfied that atmospherical air was not an unalterable thing."

Priestley was, at first, hampered in his experiments by difficulty in producing a very high temperature; eventually he solved this by obtaining a large, twelve inch, burning glass. Another technical problem — the fragility of dry glass vessels when heated — was overcome by using a gun barrel. On the 1st August, 1774 he heated "mercurius calcinatus" (red oxide of mercury) with his lens, and obtained a gas with unusual properties — "a candle burned in this air with a remarkably vigorous flame". This, clearly, required further investigation. Was it fit to breathe, for instance? He applied the best test he knew to find out whether it was wholesome or not. He had found that the gas behaved in the same way as ordinary air on the addition of "nitrous air" (nitric oxide). On the strength of this, he put a mouse into an atmosphere of the new gas, and the mouse breathed well and lived. Further experiments led Priestley to conclude that his new gas was some four to five times as good as common air. He called it dephlogisticated air — we call it oxygen.

When he used the gun barrel as a more durable container than a glass vessel he soon ran into trouble. He saturated half an ounce of lead ore with

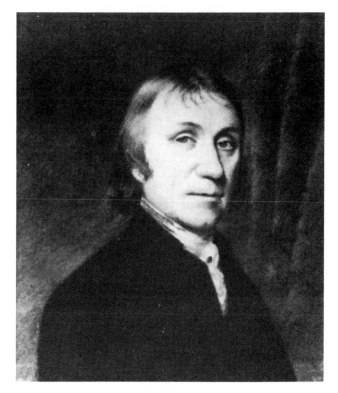

FIGURE 15
Joseph Priestley, 1733–1804.

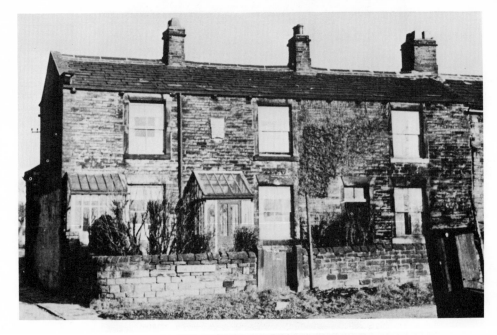

FIGURES 16 AND 17

The inscription on this house reads "Joseph Priestley, discoverer of oxygen, born on this site. A.D. 1733". It is in Owler Lane, off Fieldhead Lane, Birstall, Yorkshire. Photographs taken by Dr. Sykes, who lived about three miles away.

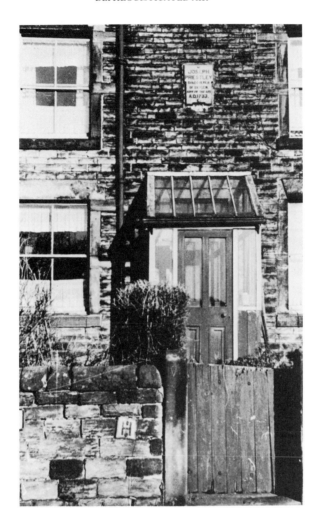

spirits of nitre, dried it, loaded it into the barrel which he then filled up to the muzzle with powdered flint.

"As soon as this mixture began to warm, air was generated very fast, insomuch that, being rather alarmed, I stood on one side; when presently there was a violent and loud explosion, by which all the contents of the gun barrel were driven out with great force, dashing to pieces the vessels that were placed to receive the air."

By a little stretch of the imagination this incident, although long before the anaesthetic era, could be described as the first anaesthetic explosion on record. We are indebted to the craftsmanship of the unknown gun-maker, that his work stood up so well to the grossly unfair test of being loaded up to the muzzle. A burst could so easily have cut short Priestley's life and work.

Priestley concluded his remarks on oxygen by suggesting that it could be used to purify the noxious air of crowded rooms, that it would magnify the force of gunpowder explosions, and that it would "augment the force of fire to a prodigious degree". He did not, apparently, try oxygen with gunpowder for himself — perhaps his first, unplanned explosion frightened him off this experiment — but he did notice that hydrogen exploded with greater violence when mixed with oxygen than with ordinary air.

He also predicted that "it might be peculiarly salutary to the lungs in certain morbid cases, when common air would not be sufficient to carry off the phlogistic putrid effluvium fast enough". As regards his own personal trial of the gas he wrote:

"My reader will not wonder, that, after having ascertained the superior goodness of dephlogisticated air by mice living in it . . . I should have the curiosity to taste it myself. I have gratified that curiosity . . . the feeling of it to my lungs was not sensibly different from that of common air; but I fancied that my breast felt peculiarly light and easy for some time afterwards. . . . Hitherto only two mice and myself have had the privilege of breathing it."

Oxygen and its properties, then, were quite well known when the anaesthetic era began. C. T. Jackson took a bag full of oxygen, with the idea that it might be used as an antidote to ether, when he witnessed an operation under ether anaesthesia at the beginning of January, 1847.[2] This was described as "the first act indicating . . . that he had any interest in the subject".

James Robinson, a dentist, of Gower Street in London, was the first man to administer ether anaesthesia in England. He used oxygen after ether anaesthesia as early as April, 1847.

"For the last week I have been using, as a means of resuscitating patients, after inhaling the vapour of ether, pure oxygen gas, with the most perfect success. Today I operated in nine cases on the teeth; to each patient I gave a full dose of the ether vapour, and subsequently a few inhalations of oxygen. In not one case did the patients complain of debility, and all recovered perfectly in less than a minute and a half, timed by the medical men present."[3]

Mr. William Hooper, about the same time, marketed an oxygen attachment for Robinson's inhaler.[4] Thomas Cattell, helpfully, suggested an easy method of making oxygen, which was not something which could be purchased at the time. He gave details of four methods for doing this.[5] One of the early articles published on oxygen as a therapeutic agent was by S. B. Birch, of London in 1859.[6,7] By this date the firm of Barth's was supplying the condensed gas in cylinders. Shortly afterwards, Benjamin Ward Richardson entered the field. He had been experimenting with animals and oxygen since 1852, and felt confident enough to make three propositions based on his observations. These were:

"The influence of pure oxygen, as an excitant, differs according to the animal; being most marked in animals of quick respiration and high temperature; and least marked or nil in those of feeble respiration and lower temperature.

"Oxygen, when breathed over and over again, although freed entirely from carbonic acid or other known products of respiration, loses its power of supporting life; the process of life ceasing, not from the introduction of a poison but by a negation, or a withdrawal of some principal extant in the primitive oxygen, which is essential to life.

"Oxygen, while it is essential to muscular irritability and muscular power, exerts its influence over muscle, not as a direct excitant of muscular contraction, but by supplying to the muscle an agent or force by which the muscle is fitted for contraction on the application of an exciting cause."[8]

Richardson, therefore, with his own closed-circuit oxygen apparatus and carbon dioxide absorption was not able to keep most of his animals alive and well for more than about ten hours.

Mr. J. Webster, of Birmingham, patented a process for the manufacture of oxygen in 1862. His apparatus consisted of an iron retort in which he distilled a mixture of sodium nitrate, or any other convenient nitrate, with an oxide of iron or zinc. The gases given off were passed through water to condense those which were not wanted and the oxygen which remained was collected in a "proper receiver".[9]

In 1863, M. Laugier told a meeting of the French Academy of Sciences of his use of oxygen baths in the treatment of incipient, senile gangrene of the limbs. *The Lancet*, recording this, added cautiously "However plausible the theory advanced may appear to be, the success of the practice remains to be demonstrated".[10] Ten years later, Dr. Léon Labbé, of Paris, described his faith in the method, and presented a case report.[11] In 1866, Dr. R. H. Goolden, of St. Thomas' Hospital in London, used oxygen inhalations in the treatment of gout and phagadaenic (chronic, eroding) ulceration with, seemingly, good effect. The patient with the chronic ulceration also had double pneumonia.[12]

The first deaths resulting from an oxygen explosion occurred in Manchester, in 1865.[13] Mr. Crowther, a dealer in oxygen and hydrogen, together with his son, were killed by the explosion of an iron retort in which oxygen was being prepared from chlorate of potash and binoxide of manganese. An analyst found soot, charcoal, or lampblack, in the mixture which would have made it as dangerous as gunpowder. A verdict of manslaughter was returned against the chemist who had sold the ingredients to the deceased. This, I think was pretty hard on him, unless he was the actual maker of the various ingredients which he sold.

An important step forward was made when it became possible to liquefy oxygen for storage. In 1877, a telegram was sent by Professor Pictet of Geneva to Professor Tyndall:

"Oxygène liquifié samedi par acides sulfureux et carboniques combinés. Pression, 320 atmosphères. Température, 100 deg. Centigrade de froid."[14]

Previously all attempts to liquefy oxygen thus had failed.

In 1890, John Chambers, who was then in Paris, but had been a practising physician in the United States of America, stressed the value of oxygen inhalation in the treatment of pneumonia. He obtained his oxygen, and recommended others to do likewise, from the laboratory of a chemist.[15] In the same year oxygen was made available commercially by Brin's Oxygen Company, of Westminster. Their product cost a fraction of that produced by more old-fashioned processes but, they were, at the time, not able to compress it into cylinders at pressures of 120 atmospheres. Nonetheless their oxygen cost from 2d. to 4d. for each cubic foot and, being extracted from atmospheric air, was entirely free of chlorine.[16]

George Foy, a surgeon in Dublin, commented in 1891 upon a recent death under chloroform which had occurred in Belfast. He observed that no mention had been made of the method of resuscitation for which, he thought, oxygen would have been useful. He concluded by saying:

"As the liquefied gas can now be readily obtained, I think a bottle of oxygen with a suitable inhalation apparatus attached should be in the operating theatre of every hospital."[17]

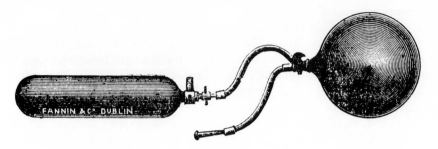

FIGURE 18

British Medical Journal, 1892, **1**, 180. George Foy's oxygen apparatus, made by Fannin and Company, of Dublin. (Thomas Beddoes pointed out that oxygen was an antidote to asphyxia.) The rubber bladder on the right was attached through a stop-cock to a cylinder of oxygen and to a vulcanite mouthpiece.

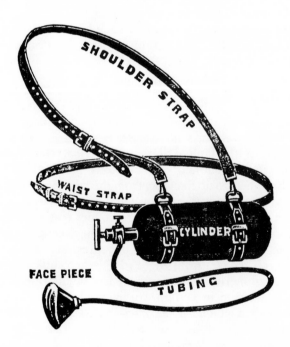

FIGURE 19

Lancet, 1896, **2**, 1314. T. B. Abbott, of Aberford. Portable oxygen apparatus, suggested after his experience of a colliery explosion at Micklefield in May, 1896. Oxygen was valuable for resuscitation, but large cylinders could not be taken over the falls of roof in the workings. Made by Reynolds and Branston, Leeds, it used a 10 cu. ft. cylinder.

George Stoker, a physician at the London Throat Hospital wrote, in 1896, on the surgical use of oxygen in the local treatment of wounds.[18] He described a box with a rubber sleeve, and other devices, to fit different parts of the body, and claimed that oxygen, applied locally, relieved pain, abolished smell and caused rapid healing in many of those cases which had failed to respond to other treatments.

In 1908, Leonard Hill and Martin Flack, both of The London Hospital, tested the effects of oxygen in athletes, one of whom they persuaded to be a co-author of their paper.[19] They found that inhalation of oxygen prior to a race enabled the athletes to better their previous performances. A few weeks later Martin Flack (who, incidentally, identified the location of the sino-auricular node in the heart) reported the attempt he had made to improve the performance of a cross-channel swimmer by giving oxygen inhalations. Flack's account is fascinating.

"In furtherance of research by us into the effects of oxygen upon the organism, I accompanied Mr. Jabez Wolffe in his attempt to swim the Channel on Saturday, September 19th. . . . The swim began at 6.6 a.m. from the Shakespeare Cliff, Dover. The swimmer was in splendid condition and in excellent spirits. He took his meals hourly. These consisted of a cup or so of Nursing Oxo with Plasmon biscuits, usually alternated with warm weak tea and sponge fingers, although on occasions Oxo would be given twice in succession, according to the swimmer's wishes. It will be noticed that there is not the amount of dextrose present in the diet that one would like to see on such an enterprise. From the very start it was obvious that Wolffe and his friends meant to 'have to go without oxygen'. The day was too good for scientific experiment, and the conditions for the swim were ideal. The weather was fine but hazy, the sea smooth, and there was little drift up and down channel. The progress made by the swimmer was extraordinary, the first fourteen miles being covered in about eight hours. The course kept was so true that the Calais packets passed quite close. On several occasions oxygen was offered, but Wolffe was so confident and going so well that its help was declined. Just before 5 o'clock it was obvious that the swimmer was far from comfortable, and then oxygen would undoubtedly have been of the utmost value. But popular opinion carried the day. Wolffe managed to get over this 'bad time', but it had told its tale. Thenceforth the progress made was not nearly so marked. The same mechanical precision of stroke was there, but its potency had gone. Soon after six the swimmer began to get anxious and asked to be accompanied by the pilot (Captain Birchfield) in the small boat. Up till then he had been accompanied in the water at frequent intervals by his friend Kellingley. From now on fatigue symptoms began to manifest themselves with increasing force, but the swimmer plodded manfully on. At 7.45, when he would undoubtedly have given up, any aid that oxygen could give was accepted. The apparatus was lowered into the small boat and taken out to the swimmer. He was now showing manifest nervous symptoms; his breathing was very laboured;

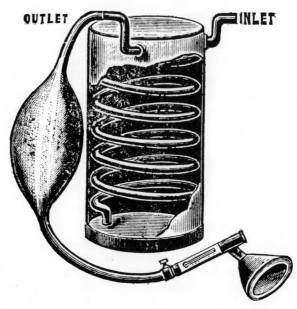

FIGURE 20

British Medical Journal, 1896, **2**, 1786. H. J. Robson described this warm oxygen apparatus which was made by Reynolds and Branston of Leeds. The cold oxygen issuing from a cylinder could be passed through this device to warm it up; the copper cylinder was placed in a basin of hot water. There is a thermometer in the glass tube near the facepiece.

his muscles were doing but little efficient work; altogether he was very 'done'. The oxygen was administered through a long rubber tube leading to a mouthpiece with inlet and outlet valves. Close to the cylinder a large rubber bag was interposed so that the amount of gas coming from the cylinder could be gauged. The pilot held the mouthpiece to the swimmer while M.F. manipulated the cylinder and watched the effect of the gas. This was, to say the least, somewhat striking. The effect of a dyspnoeic 51-in. chested man at the end of a tube of oxygen is perhaps not easily appreciated at first. The bag was emptied with such amazing rapidity and completeness that a leak seemed probable, and a big one too. A leak indeed there was, but careful inspection showed that it was only into the alveoli of an oxygen-starved man. Gradually the breathing quietened, the pressure of gas had to be reduced to less than half, and after about four minutes the swimmer quietly turned away from the tube and started swimming again in a resolute fashion. For the time being nervous symptoms had gone, dyspnoea was relieved, and the swimmer was again doing good, efficient work. The general improvement was manifest to all, but especially so to the occupants of the small boat. Oxygen was now administered about every quarter of an hour. During this time the progress was good, the tide being favourable. Unfortunately, when about a quarter of a mile from the shore

Wolffe complained of the cold, and shortly after he turned on his chest with extended limbs. The muscles were overburdened with fatigue products, and, together with the effect of cold, brought about the final collapse. The 'cramp' was not tonic, and did not persist. When we got aboard the effect of the oxygen was still wonderfully manifest. The pulse showed that the circulation was good, there was no dyspnoea, the muscles only had gone, and the swimmer was in no danger. After a few minutes' rubbing with paraffin Wolffe was on his legs, rubbing himself down with a towel. Shortly afterwards he was peacefully sleeping in his bunk after a parting dose of O_2."[20]

Professors Lazarus and Saubermann, from Berlin, described an apparatus which was an oxygen cylinder enclosing a source of radium emanation.[21] What, exactly, this was used for is not at all clear. In 1912, Leonard Hill stated flatly that the method of giving oxygen by a funnel held more or less near the patient's face was useless, and described a mask

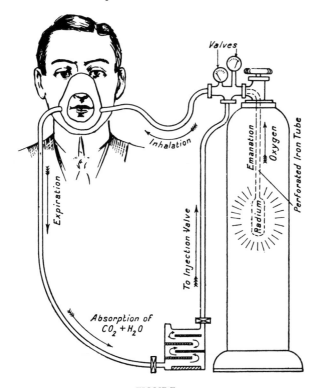

FIGURE 21
Medical Annual, 1913, 436. Professor Paul Lazarus and Professor Sauberman described this apparatus for the inhalation of radium emanation and oxygen in a closed circuit.

which a patient could easily and efficiently apply to his face. He noted that cases of pneumonia in places of high altitude and low oxygen tension, such as Mexico City, improved markedly when moved to the plains far below.[22] Sixteen years later, R. Hilton, of the Medical Unit at Bart's, said that a flow of oxygen, emitted from a funnel held 10 cms. or more from the patient's face had no effect at all, but if the funnel was pressed close a flow of one and a half litres would raise the alveolar oxygen content by 50 per cent. and a flow of 3 litres would double it.[23]

A method of administering oxygen subcutaneously was first described in 1900 and had been used, apparently with benefit, in a whole variety of conditions.[24] Dr. John McCrae, of Montreal, spoke favourably of the method,[25] and Drs. Howitt and Jones recommended it in the treatment of tetanus on the grounds that the causative organism is an obligatory anaerobe.[26] J. D. Mortimer, an anaesthetist at the Royal Waterloo Hospital in London, suggested its use for the treatment of soldiers who had been gassed. The use of gas was then a novelty, and the method was tried, and found to be useful.[27] Subcutaneous oxygen was used by T. S. Kirk in cases of pneumonia and for the treatment of burns.[28] There was no need, he said, to measure the amount of gas precisely, or to filter or warm it. As a rough

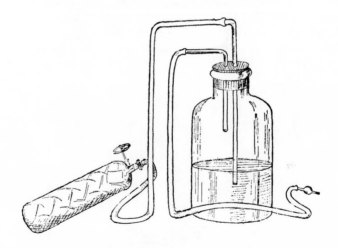

FIGURE 22
British Medical Journal, 1917, **1**, 511. H. Oswald Smith described the use of injections of oxygen in the treatment of trench foot. Oxygen, it was said, helped drive out serum through puncture holes made for the purpose, relieved pressure on blood vessels and lymphatics, and abolished the pain at once.

In 1930, Allen and Hanbury's were advertising Dr. Bayeux's oxygenator for the hypodermic administration of oxygen, using a platinum needle.

measure he suggested that 200 mls. would inflate an area equal to the palms of two hands.

J. Argyll Campbell, who did much work on oxygen inhalation, criticised the subcutaneous injection of oxygen, mainly because the amount it was possible to give in this way was far too small to be of any use.[29] As the average man consumes, at rest, 250 mls. of oxygen each minute he could see no point in giving another 250 mls. perhaps twice a day, which is 1440 minutes. Later, he reiterated this argument and calculated that if 500 mls. of oxygen were injected, and slowly absorbed over two days, then the rate of absorption would be just 0·18 mls. per minute, or just over 10 mls. per hour.[30] During that hour 15,000 mls. of oxygen would be required by a body at rest.

Several investigators began to explore the potentialities of intravenous injections of oxygen. F. W. Tunnicliffe and G. F. Stebbing stated that oxygen could be given by this route at the rate of between 600 to 1200 mls. an hour.[31] I. Singh, in 1935, reported that intravenous oxygen could supply the whole requirements of an animal if it was given in a chamber pressurised to three atmospheres.[32] He admitted, however, that there would be a risk of pulmonary embolism if the gas was given too quickly. Five years later he and a colleague in Bombay claimed that from 10 to 20 mls. could be given each minute to man. They had used this method in 6 cases and were able to supply about one tenth of the basal requirements. The method was, they pointed out, the only one by which any useful quantity of oxygen could be given by an extra-pulmonary route.[33]

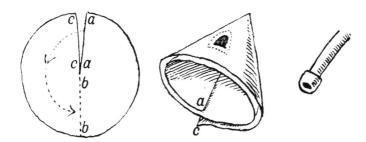

FIGURE 23

Lancet, 1931, **1**, 701. W. E. Waller described his improvisation for giving oxygen in private practice. A 10 inch diameter circle is cut from several layers of newspapers and a single radial cut is made through all the layers. The paper is then folded, as shown, to make a cone which is kept in shape by sewing the free edges in place, or with safety pins. A hole is cut at the apex for the oxygen delivery tube to enter, this tube being secured by a flange. A small D-shaped opening is cut out of the mask and a simple valve made by covering this with a flap of tissue paper gummed down on its straight edge only. The edges of the mask are then cut to fit the face.

In 1944 Dr. Frederick Viedge asked "Would not the bone marrow offer a convenient site for the direct administration of oxygen gas?" Nothing much seems to have come of this, and Viedge merely said "If this suggestion has any originality and any value I leave it to more capable hands than mine to initiate."[34]

Henry A. Ellis, of Middlesbrough, made a far-reaching claim in 1920 when he said that oxygen prepared in different ways had different effects.[35] He claimed that oxygen prepared from chlorate of potash and manganese dioxide was contaminated with chlorine, and this "chlorine oxygen" was both a hypnotic and a stimulant. "It was sufficiently powerful to make the attendant find it difficult to keep awake in such an atmosphere." Oxygen stored in a cylinder, he said, was "dead oxygen" since it possessed no properties other than that of eliminating oxygen lack. The third form he had tried, prepared from water and sodium dioxide, "sodium oxygen", improved metabolism and, in cases of phthisis, made the muscles more resilient. He believed this last form of oxygen to be of greatest value.

J. Argyll Campbell, referring to oxygen convulsions, said that these were first reported by Paul Bert in 1878 in animals breathing oxygen at several atmospheres' pressure. Campbell found that, under these conditions, plasma alone contained enough dissolved oxygen for the needs of the body when at rest.[36] The convulsions developed more rapidly if the animals were given a 5% carbon dioxide mixture with oxygen under pressure. In 1938, a leading article in the *British Medical Journal* stated that mammals cannot live continuously in regions where there is 10% of oxygen, or less, in the atmosphere. This corresponds with an altitude of 20,000 feet above sea level. This limit, first established in animals in a laboratory, was confirmed in a study of sulphur miners in the Andes who could not keep healthy if they lived and slept at above 17,500 feet; they were, however, able to work, slowly, at 19,000 feet. Their camp at 17,500 feet above sea level was believed to be the highest in existence, but the people living there descended to 12,000 feet for confinements and "a proper game of football".[37]

Liquid oxygen storage for hospital use, instead of huge numbers of cylinders, seem first to have been suggested in 1940, and was the subject of a note in *The Lancet* of that year.[38] This recorded that "It is doubtful whether more than 10 per cent. of hospitals in this country are properly equipped for oxygen therapy, and indeed, owing to the efficiency of some of the commercial services, better conditions can often be secured in the patient's home than in Hospital." A few months later, a French hospital installed the necessary equipment for a liquid oxygen store.[39]

The more disastrous effects of inhaling high oxygen tensions for long

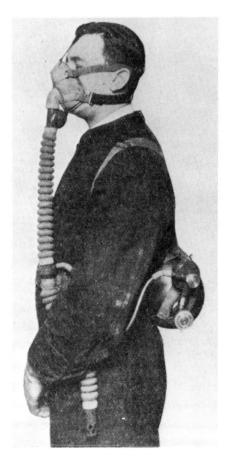

FIGURES 24 AND 25

Lancet, 1934, **2**, 1122. Raymond Greene. The Everest oxygen apparatus for the 1933 expedition. Made by Siebe, Gorman and Company. Light weight R.A.F. oxygen cylinders were used, and the apparatus weighed 12 lbs. 12 ozs. It was to be used only for the final 200 feet of the ascent.

The apparatus was tested in low pressure and low temperature chambers. The upper part of the wide tube acted as a rebreathing bag to collect oxygen during expiration, and prevented waste.

Figure 25 is on page 78.

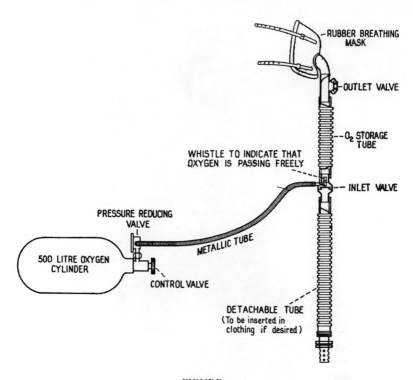

FIGURE 25

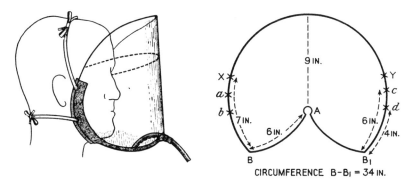

CIRCUMFERENCE B-B₁ = 34 IN.

FIGURE 26

Lancet, 1940, **1**, 648. Alice Rose and Thomas Holmes Sellors described this improvised oxygen mask which was made of light plastic or X-ray film. The edges AB and AB₁ were sewn together and a piece of copper wire oversewn along XBAB₁Y. Tapes were stitched on at a, b, c and d and rubber tubing from the oxygen source is inserted through the apex of the cone and fixed with stitches inside the mask. This part of the tube had holes cut in its length. The edges of the mask next to the patient's face were padded with lint. It was claimed that a flow of 3 litres a minute could give up to 40% oxygen in the alveoli; a six litre flow gave up to 50% enrichment.

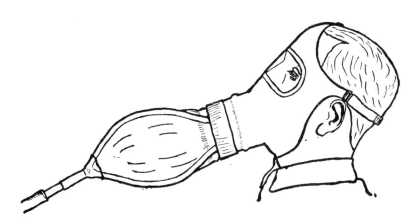

FIGURE 27

British Medical Journal, 1940, **2**, 519. H. L. Marriott described this adaptation of the civilian gas mask as an emergency oxygen apparatus. A rubber football bladder with a hole cut in it was stretched over the canister of the mask, and oxygen entered at the other end of the bladder. An expiratory valve was not needed with this form of gas mask. Expiration took place between the edge of the mask and the face, but there was no air leak during inspiration as the rubber mask moulded itself directly to the wearer's face.

periods of time were not reported until 1942, when T. L. Terry described retro-lental fibroplasia in babies given indiscriminate oxygen therapy.[40] This was one hundred and sixty-eight years after Joseph Priestley and his two mice had the "privilege" of first inhaling the gas. Probably, it was not until the 1940s that oxygen adminstration reached such a reasonable pitch of efficiency that it was possible, under certain conditions, to give an overdose of a vital and, ordinarily, innocuous gas.

REFERENCES

[1] Priestley, J. (1775) *Experiments and Observations on Different Kinds of Air.* London: J. Johnson.

[2] Statements, supported by evidence, of Wm. T. G. Morton on his claim to the discovery of anaesthetic ether, submitted to the Select Committee appointed by the Senate of the United States. Jan. 21., 1853. Washington.

[3] Robinson, J. (1847) A mode of resuscitating patients after inhaling the vapour of ether. *Lancet*, 1, 371.

[4] Hooper, W. (1847) Inhalation of oxygen for resuscitating etherised patients. *Pharmaceutical Journal*, 6, 508–509.

[5] Cattell, T. (1847) On oxygen, as a corrective of the secondary effects of ether in surgical operations. *Lancet*, 1, 422.

[6] Birch, S. B. (1859) On oxygen as a therapeutic agent. *British Medical Journal*, 2, 1033–1035.

[7] Birch, S. B. (1859) On oxygen as a therapeutic agent. *British Medical Journal*, 2, 1053–1055.

[8] Richardson, B. W. (1860) On the process of oxygenation in animal bodies. *British Medical Journal*, 2, 549–550.

[9] Annotation (1862) Manufacture of oxygen gas. *Lancet*, 1, 560.

[10] Annotation (1863) Baths of oxygen gas. *Lancet*, 1, 706.

[11] Annotation (1873) Senile gangrene of the foot cured by the oxygen bath. *Lancet*, 2, 152.

[12] Goolden, R. H. (1866) Treatment of disease by oxygen. *Lancet*, 1, 270–271.

[13] Annotation (1865) Fatal explosion. *British Medical Journal*, 1, 24.

[14] Annotation (1877) Liquefaction of oxygen. *British Medical Journal*, 2, 931.

[15] Chambers, J. (1890) Oxygen gas in pneumonia. *Lancet*, 1, 1120–1121.

[16] Annotation (1890) The production of oxygen gas. *Lancet*, 1, 1407.

[17] Foy, G. (1891) Death under chloroform. *Lancet*, 1, 1340.

[18] Stoker, G. (1896) The surgical uses of oxygen gas. *British Medical Journal*, 2, 1208–1212.

[19] Hill, L., Flack, M. & Just, T. H. (1908) The influence of oxygen inhalations on athletes. *British Medical Journal*, 2, 499–500.

[20] Flack, M. (1908) The effect of Oxygen on Wolffe in his Channel Swim of September 19th. *British Medical Journal*, 2, 968.

[21] Saubermann, S. (1911) Radium emanation and physiological processes. *British Medical Journal*, 2, 914–916.

[22] Hill, L. (1912) The administration of oxygen. *British Medical Journal*, 1, 71–72.

[23] Hilton, R. (1928) A comparison of the efficiency of some methods of oxygen administration. *British Medical Journal*, 1, 441–442.

[24] Anonymous (1915) Hypodermic injections of oxygen gas in therapeutics. *British Medical Journal*, 1, 973–974.

[25] Annotation (1915) The subcutaneous injection of oxygen. *Lancet*, 1, 32.

[26] Howitt, H. O., Jones, D. H. (1915) Injection of oxygen as a treatment for tetanus. *Lancet*, 1, 752–753.

[27] Mortimer, J. D. (1915) Poisonous gases. *British Medical Journal*, **1**, 1027–1028.

[28] Kirk, T. S. (1928) Use of subcutaneous injections of oxygen. *British Medical Journal*, **2**, 195–196.

[29] Campbell, J. A. (1928) Uses of subcutaneous injections of oxygen. *British Medical Journal*, **2**, 274.

[30] Campbell, J. A. (1932) Subcutaneous injection of oxygen. *British Medical Journal*, **2**, 274.

[31] Tunnicliffe, F. W., Stebbing, G. F. (1916) The intravenous injection of oxygen as a therapeutic measure. *Lancet*, **2**, 321–323.

[32] Annotation. (1935) Life without breathing. *Lancet*, **2**, 380.

[33] Singh, I., Shah, M. J. (1940) Intravenous injection of oxygen under normal atmospheric pressure. *Lancet*, **1**, 922–923.

[34] Viedge, F. (1944) Oxygen via bone-marrow? *British Medical Journal*, **2**, 876.

[35] Ellis, H. A. (1920) The therapeutic uses of oxygen. *Lancet*, **1**, 569.

[36] Campbell, J. A. (1934) Oxygen convulsions. *Lancet*, **1**, 105–106.

[37] Editorial (1938) Oxygen want and oxygen therapy. *British Medical Journal*, **1**, 235–236.

[38] Annotation (1940) Pros and cons of liquid oxygen. *Lancet*, **1**, 842.

[39] Annotation (1940) Liquid oxygen in Hospital Practice. *British Medical Journal*, **2**, 142.

[40] Terry, T. L. (1942) Extreme prematurity and fibroblastic overgrowth of persistent vascular sheath behind each crystalline lens. *American Journal of Ophthalmology*, **25**, 203–204.

CHAPTER 7

THE PIONEER OF INTRAVENOUS ANAESTHESIA

Most histories of anaesthesia refer to Oré, of Bordeaux, and his use of intravenous chloral, but they seem only to mention his name in passing and give no details of his work. I wanted to discover more about Oré and his researches, for his idea was a very original one at the time.

I found, first of all, that he had written a book entitled *Études cliniques sur l'anesthésie chirurgicale par la méthode des injections de chloral dans les veines* which was published in Paris in 1875.[1] It was an elusive book, and quite difficult to find but, eventually, I obtained a copy from the Bibliothèque Nationale in Paris. It was a green, paper-backed book of 154 pages, with two plates, one of them in colour. Dr. Oré, who rarely mentioned his christian name (which was Pierre-Cyprien) was Professor of Physiology at the School of Medicine and Honorary Surgeon to the Hospitals of Bordeaux.

He began his book by pointing out that he had addressed two memoirs on his subject to the Académie des Sciences in 1873 and, based on these, he intended to divide his book into two parts.

"In the first I will demonstrate that, looked at from the point of view of pure experimental physiology, the intravenous injection of chloral constitutes a means of producing anaesthesia superior to all others. In the second I will report all the facts on which anaesthesia has been happily produced by this method in man, and compare chloral narcosis [*l'insensibilité chloralique*] with that caused by ether and chloroform, and endeavour to prove the superiority of the first over the other."

The first part of the book gives three sample descriptions of animal experiments after which Oré refers his readers to his previously published work for a fuller account. He concluded that intravenous chloral was the most powerful of all the anaesthetics then available.

"A terrier dog weighing 7 Kg. was given 2 Gm. of chloral intravenously. Twenty seconds after the completion of the injection the animal fell into a profound sleep. Sensibility was almost completely abolished; but there were still signs of pain on pinching the ears or paws forcibly. This lasted only a short time; for five minutes later neither punctures, nor deep incisions, nor twisting, nor the actual cautery gave rise to the least sign of pain. The temperature fell by 2 degrees, but the respiration was regular."

Chloral given intravenously, he continues, gave a constancy and duration of effect which is lacking when the same substance is given by

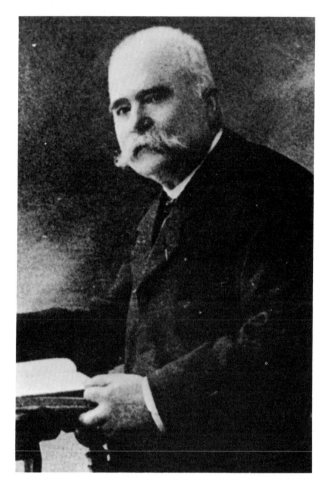

FIGURE 28
Dr. Pierre Cyprien Oré (1828–1889)

mouth or hypodermically. It gave complete insensibility to all stimuli, and the dose required to produce this result varied with the weight of the animal. A dose of 2 Gm. could safely be given to a dog weighing 7 Kg. and one weighing 20 Kg. could receive 7 Gm. The duration of anaesthesia varied from 1 to 5 hours; it then ceased, but the animal was depressed for the following 24 hours, or more. There was never any trouble with the animals' respiration so long as the dose used was not absolutely poisonous.

In the second part of his book, Dr. Oré describes his use of the method in man, and gives detailed accounts of 36 cases. The chloral solution which he used was specially prepared for him by Monsieur le pharmacien L. Begein.

Like all innovations, Oré's method aroused opposition.

"Is it rational, writes Monsieur Fano in his indignant fervour, to submit to such experiments a patient who is to be operated upon for cataract, like that done at Bordeaux? I read lately in a medical journal of one of our Parisian confrères having performed an intravenous injection in a dog in Britain . . . and has been arraigned before a court by the English society for the protection of animals and that, while escaping a conviction, the court at Norwich blamed his conduct. If a society existed for the protection of man, what court would exonerate a surgeon from having made an intravenous injection of chloral in order to operate for cataract?"

To this criticism Oré made a four page reply and quoted many witnesses to the benefits of chloral anaesthesia in eye surgery, including the famous ophthalmologist von Graefe. He concluded:

"Anaesthesia by the intravenous injection of chloral fulfils the desires of the oculists; with it their ideal is attained. It gives rapid and absolute insensibility of the cornea, without nausea and without reflex movements. *'On opère comme sur le cadavre'*."

Oré was in the habit of giving the injection of chloral fairly slowly. In one case, selected at random from his series, the patient was sleepy after the injection of 4 Gm. over 6 minutes, and his speech was confused. At the end of the next minute, during which a further 1·5 Gm. were given, speech became even more confused and the patient was apathetic. 11 minutes after the injection began, during which time 7·5 Gm. had been given, sleep occurred, but the cornea was still sensitive. A total dose of 8 Gm. given over a period of 12 minutes produced complete insensibility.

His list of thirty-six cases included about ten eye operations, one ovarian cyst (which died on the operating table from haemorrhage), castration, tumours of the breast, thigh amputations and a resection of a knee joint. A thirty-seventh case is added as a post-script. One of the cataract cases, a

ÉTUDES CLINIQUES

SUR

L'ANESTHÉSIE CHIRURGICALE

PAR LA MÉTHODE

DES INJECTIONS DE CHLORAL DANS LES VEINES

Par le **Dʳ ORÉ**

Lauréat de l'Institut, Chirurgien honoraire des Hôpitaux,

Docteur ès-Sciences naturelles,

Professeur de Physiologie et Lauréat de l'École de Médecine de Bordeaux,

Membre et Lauréat de l'Académie des Sciences (Médaille d'argent et Médaille d'or) ;

Membre honoraire de la Société de Médecine de Gand ; Associé national de la Société d'Anthropologie ;

Correspondant de la Société de Chirurgie, de la Société de Biologie,

de la Société des Sciences, Lettres et Arts d'Évreux,

des Sociétés de Médecine de Marseille, Caen, Metz, Poitiers ; de la Société de Médecine

et de Chirurgie pratique de Montpellier ; Officier de l'Instruction publique ; Chevalier de la Légion d'honneur

et de l'Ordre de la Conception du Portugal.

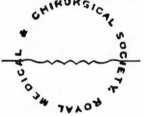

PARIS

J.-B. BAILLIÈRE et FILS

LIBRAIRES-ÉDITEURS DE L'ACADÉMIE DE MÉDECINE

16, rue Hautefeuille, 16

—

1875

FIGURE 29

The title page of Dr. Oré's book.

woman of 60 years old, is of interest. Four years previously she had a carcinoma of the breast to be removed and all attempts to anaesthetise her with chloroform failed. Chloroform, from three different sources was used for no less than two hours; it was given on a sponge enveloped in a cornet of stiff paper, and also on a compress. The patient, says Oré, was "*absolument refractaire*". It sounds inconceivable that a woman, elderly at that, should resist chloroform if it was properly administered. It is far more likely that this inhalational anaesthetic was badly and timidly given. After all, there were no specialist anaesthetists in Europe in those days or, indeed for many years afterwards. The resulting poor general anaesthesia by inhalation was probably one of the main reasons why so many injection methods were developed on the Continent. Anyway, this lady's anaesthetic with chloroform was abandoned after two hours and her operation carried out without anaesthesia. Then, four years later, she had to have bilateral cataracts removed.

"She wished to see again . . . One thing only delayed her decision to be operated upon; she was frightened of the pain and she knew by experience that she could not count on chloroform. We reassured her and made her understand that another method could make her insensible. It was a magnificent occasion to establish on the same person a comparison between inhalational and intravenous anaesthesia. We could establish, on the same patient, the power of the two methods. And so, within 12 minutes 45 seconds, 8 Gm. of chloral injected into the veins of this lady, so resistant to the action of chloroform, had produced complete anaesthesia which lasted 15 minutes. To us, comment on this seems superfluous. The insensibility of the eye was complete; we were operating as if on a corpse."

Another of the cataract cases had an unfortunate ending, and it was the only one in which death could be attributed to the chloral. A man of 45, with no disease of his heart or lungs, had bilateral cataracts. He was pallid and "Not endowed with great vital energy". After 6 Gm. had been injected, over 6 minutes and 15 seconds, the cornea became insensible and the right cataract was removed. This took about two minutes, during which the pulse rose from 112 to 160. As the left eye was about to be dealt with it was noticed that the circulation and respiration were failing. One of the terminals of an electric machine was applied to the epigastrium, and the other placed over the course of the vagus and phrenic nerves. The patient's condition improved but, unfortunately, the electricity got weaker and weaker and then faded completely; the patient died. This was before the days of mains electricity; the machine must have been powered by batteries which had been allowed to run down.

Both here and elsewhere in the book Oré states that electricity is the one antidote to chloral anaesthesia. When describing the apparatus required he says that an electrical machine, in good working order, is absolutely essential — just as necessary as the syringe used for injection. Later, he wrote:

"The electric current is the best means to combat anaesthesia produced by chloral. It stops it rapidly and brings back sensibility and movements. All stimuli, even the most energetic, are incapable of bringing about the least sign of sensibility in animals under chloral; the electric current alone makes it immediately re-appear. Is not one entitled to find in this fact a new proof of the analogy which exists between electric and nervous action?"

Objections had been made that the method would lead to phlebitis. Oré had never seen this in animals, and only once in man in 65 cases. (Here, he was relying on the experience of others who had used his technique, as well as on his own observations.) It was also said that the injection would cause clotting of the blood. Oré had never seen this happen, even after repeated injections. In one case, of rabies, 33 Gm. of chloral were given in 24 hours without thrombosis; in a case of tetanus there was no clotting after 9 injections.

Oré summed up the advantages of his method as follows. The injections did not affect respiration, never caused a stage of excitation and were never accompanied by vomiting. They gave an insensibility, the duration of which varied with the dose and had, in his cases, been 45 minutes. They were always followed by calm, deep, regular sleep lasting, on average, for 20 hours as a consequence of which the patients escaped the otherwise inevitable, post-operative pain. The injections, when properly performed, were never accompanied by phlebitis or clotting. As for haematuria, which had also been mentioned as a complication, this only showed itself rarely and had, so far, been a phenomenon of no practical importance. In all cases in which clots or phlebitis had occurred, if the cause was looked for it would be found to be due to the way in which the chloral had been given or to some previous alteration in the blood, and never to the drug itself.

"These conditions show, without it being necessary to emphasise it, the superiority of chloral anaesthesia over other anaesthetics, particularly chloroform, the danger of which is more appreciated the better one knows it."

The duration of injection, in Oré's cases, averaged $11\frac{1}{2}$ minutes, the average dose was $7\frac{1}{2}$ Gm. and the average duration of anaesthesia was about 45 minutes. The total duration of "*l'influence chloralique*" was 22 hours.

Oré's summary of the advantages of his method was far too dogmatic,

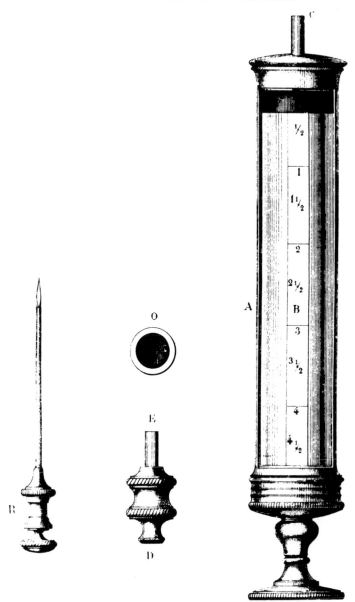

FIGURE 30

Oré's syringe and needle. When full the syringe contained 5 Grams of chloral in distilled water; the graduations on the plunger indicated how much chloral had been injected. The short, stubby connector, which contained a metallic sieve, was placed between the syringe and the needle. Oré's needle was made of gold.

89

considering his small number of cases. Words like "always" and "never" should certainly not be used when arguing from a series of just 36 cases.

He also reported a case of tetanus treated with almost 27 Gm. of chloral given by mouth. The patient died and, at post mortem, the chloral was seen to have had a caustic, vesicant action on the gastric mucosa, and this had lead to widespread lesions in the stomach.

Oré's description of the administration of intravenous chloral begins by stating that two instruments are essential — a convenient syringe and an electrical apparatus. The original model of Pravaz's syringe, he had found, was liable to transfix the vein and the solution would then be injected perivenously. His own modification was easily detachable and was only fitted to the needle when the latter was safely positioned in the vein. The barrel of his syringe contained 5 Gm. of chloral diluted in 17 mls. of distilled water. The piston rod was marked with numbered divisions indicating the number of Grams of chloral it contained. The syringe itself fitted a connector which contained a fine sieve or filter, and the connector, in turn, fitted on to the intravenous cannula which was made of gold. The original plate in Oré's book stated that it was the exact size of the syringe which means therefore, that the cannula, with its stilette, was two and a half inches long.

Oré stressed the fact that the puncture of the vein should be made without its prior dissection or isolation although, in fat subjects, a simple incision in the skin over the vein could be made provided that no further dissection took place. He was, of course, writing in the very early days of antiseptic surgery and he may, perhaps, have made his stipulation to reduce the risk of infection. The validity of Lister's suggestions had yet to be generally recognised. In the description of the syringe, and of how it should be used, no hint is given of surgical cleanliness or antisepsis. It is very probable that the syringe was brought out and used just as it was and without any preparation whatsoever.

Pierre-Cyprien Oré retired from his post as surgeon to the Saint André Hospital, Bordeaux on the 31st December, 1874 and this put an end to his opportunities for further research. However, two doctors at the University of Ghent, M. V. Deneffe and A. Van Wetter took up the idea and "the new anaesthetic method . . . replaced chloroform at the Ghent hospital". They wrote two books on the subject[2,3] which were published 1875 and 1876 in Brussels. They clearly thought highly of their work. The 1875 copy now in the library of The Wellcome Institute for the History of Medicine, in London, was that presented by the two authors to the King of Holland and bears the inscription "*À Sa Majesté Le Roi de Hollande. Hommage de ses très humbles et très obeissants serviteurs, V. Deneffe. Aug. Van Wetter.*"

The disadvantages of Oré's method are twofold. The dangers of intravenous injection without asepsis or antisepsis would be certain to have led to trouble sooner or later, although it does not seem to have done so in his small series. This was sheer luck. The second danger was from the slow, prolonged excretion of chloral from the body, a disadvantage it shared with hedonal, another long-lasting (and short-lived) anaesthetic given in the same way nearly forty years later. The very prolonged after-sleep due to this slow excretion would have become a potent source of respiratory complications after major surgery.

Not until the coming of the ultra-short acting barbiturates, some 60 years after his initial experiments, did Oré's revolutionary method come into general use. Pierre-Cyprien Oré, of Bordeaux, deserves remembrance for his brilliant idea which was born before its time.

REFERENCES

[1] Oré, P–C. (1875) *Études cliniques sur l'anesthésie chirurgicale par la méthode des injections de chloral dans les veines.* Paris, J. B. Baillière et Fils.

[2] Deneffe, V., Van Wetter, A. (1875) *De l'anesthésie produite par injection intra-veineuse de Chloral.* Brussels, Libraire de Henri Manceaux.

[3] Deneffe, V., Van Wetter, A. (1876) *Nouvelles études sur l'anesthésie par injection intra-veineuse de chloral selon la méthode de M. Le Professeur Oré.* Brussels, Libraire de Henri Manceaux.

CHAPTER 8

THE ALL-IMPORTANT AIRWAY

When general anaesthesia, as we know it, was born — at the Massachusetts General Hospital on the 16th October, 1846[1] — there was little need to safeguard the airway. The narcosis was usually so light that the cough and swallowing reflexes were still active and the muscles were never relaxed enough to allow the jaw or the tongue to fall back and obstruct respiration. For example, Mr. J. G. Lansdown removed a leg by amputation through the thigh at the Bristol General Hospital in January, 1847,[2] less than three weeks after the arrival of the great news in England. The ether was given by Mr. Herapath, and the administration was said to be quite successful. Its depth can be judged by the fact that wine was given at intervals during the operation; this seems to have been a fairly common practice in these early days. Similarly, J. Mason Warren, one of the surgeons at the Massachusetts General who had witnessed Morton's first public demonstration of ether anaesthesia, described how, soon afterwards, Morton had etherised a Mr. Hathaway for an operation on his hand.

"Very soon after the operation had commenced, he recovered his consciousness sufficiently to inquire how we were getting on, requesting that we should not hurry, but that the operation should be done thoroughly. This being completed, and the wound dressed, he said that he had been well aware during the greater portion of the time of what we were doing, but felt no more pain than he would have experienced from an ordinary examination of the part."[3]

It soon became apparent, however, that there were difficulties and dangers, especially in operations upon or near the mouth, throat and nose. These problems were dealt with in a variety of ways. George Hayward who, on the day after "Ether Day," operated on the second case anaesthetised by Morton for the removal of a fatty tumour from an arm refused, for a time, to publicise the use of Morton's "Letheon" unless he was told what it was, having no liking for secret remedies. Morton, eventually, agreed to draw aside the veil of secrecy surrounding his new agent and, having done so, ensured the enthusiastic use of ether anaesthesia at the Massachusetts General Hospital. On November 7th 1846 Dr. John Collins Warren operated to remove part of a lower jaw. This was the first time that surgeon and the anaesthetist wished to use the same territory at the same time. George Hayward's comment on the anaesthetic was:

". . . sensibility was in some measure restored before it [the operation] was over, and from the situation of the part operated upon, it was of course impossible to allow the patient to inhale the ether a second time."[4]

This was merely three weeks after ether was first used in Boston and there simply had not been time or experience enough to attempt to cope with the problems presented by this formidable case. All Morton could do was to put the patient lightly under, for the day of deep anaesthesia had not yet dawned, and then stand aside for the surgeon to begin. Quickly as the surgery was performed, the light anaesthesia wore off still more quickly. At least the patient had the benefit of being unconscious for the first part of the operation.

Other surgeons solved the problem by dodging it altogether. James Syme, in Edinburgh, always insisted on having unskilled students to give chloroform by a standardised, crude and simple method which was quite unsuitable for these difficult cases. He abandoned the idea of providing anaesthesia for these unfortunates, and simply operated without it in the old, brutal way. There was some excuse for this at first, but he continued this barbarous, and unnecessary, practice for at least seventeen years,[5] in spite of the fact that the first solution to the difficulty had been produced by John Snow all of fourteen years earlier in a patient in the recumbent posture.[6] He preferred, however, to anaesthetise these patients sitting up and to keep the level of anaesthesia so light that the cough reflex was still present (although he was one of the few men who had the knowledge and experience to produce deep anaesthesia when required). Snow also tilted the patient's head forward from time to time to empty the accumulated blood from the throat. He administered chloroform successfully for the excision of a jaw as early as 1849 by this technique.[7] The method had a very long life, which indicated that it could be safe and reasonably satisfactory in skilled hands. Fifty-three years later, Alexander Wilson and Mr. Whitehead, of Manchester, described its essential principles again and illustrated the "rocking chair method".[8]

James Miller was Professor of Systematic Surgery at Edinburgh while Syme held the Chair of Clinical Surgery and it was he who, in 1847, removed the necrosed radius of a child, the first patient to be operated upon at the Edinburgh Royal Infirmary under chloroform anaesthesia, which was administered by James Simpson.[9] Miller went on to use chloroform himself and used a simple and crude method of administration, similar to Syme's, and also ran into trouble. He wrote a text-book of surgery[10] in 1850 and added a lengthy appendix entitled "Surgical Experience of Chloroform", which makes this quite clear.

"In operations on the mouth and nose, anaesthesia must be used warily, if at all.

"The obvious and urgent cause of prudence here is the risk of asphyxia by blood escaping into the air-passages . . . in the deep stupor of Surgical Anaesthesia the patient . . . is alike dull to swallow or to cough . . . Operating once for cancer of the nose . . . I began with anaesthesia. From the track of the scalpel blood burst forth in large quantity; and, although I had arranged the patient in a sitting posture, I soon found that he was placed in imminent jeopardy of his life. The blood actually boiled and gurgled in his throat; and I was glad to find that consciousness speedily returned . . . I had to wait until the anaesthesia had passed wholly off . . . and then completed a bloody and painful, but safe operation.

"In operating for polypus of the nose, I have employed chloroform; but always took care to have the patient seated very erect, and ever and anon to have the head

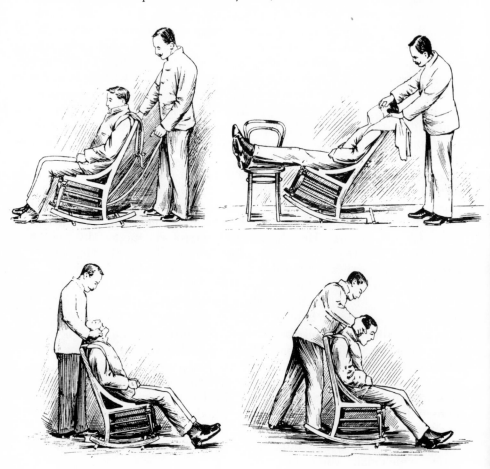

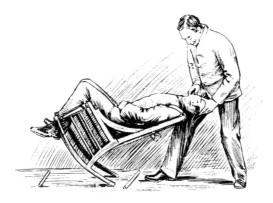

FIGURE 31
Alexander Wilson, of Manchester, described the various position his patients adopted
during Whitehead's operation for excision of the tongue in *The Medical Annual* of 1904
(page 692). The patient was secured, as in the first picture, to a rocking chair by means
of a roller towel. The second picture shows the position of the patient during the
induction of anaesthesia, and the third depicts the position of the patient during the
operation. The fourth picture shows the position adopted whenever the patient's mouth
and pharynx had to be cleared of blood, etc., and the final picture shows the patient
thrown back into the horizontal position whenever the signs of syncope appeared.

stooped forwards so as to get the mouth and throat cleared of blood...
notwithstanding the latter precaution a good deal of blood has reached the stomach,
with perhaps a polypus or two from the posterior fauces; but I have never been
troubled by the entry of either into the air-passages... it is obvious that if
chloroform be employed in operations on the mouth or nose, it must be used very
cautiously. The patient is laid recumbent during the administration; for that
posture, as formerly stated, is very favourable to the desired result being rapidly
and satisfactorily obtained. In operating, the position must be changed to that of
sitting; or the patient is arranged on his side, so as to make the orifice of the mouth
dependent."

"A much respected friend ... fond of the healing art, but not professing even
a knowledge of it, mourns the comparative exclusion of such cases from the benefits
of anaesthesia. 'It cannot be true', says he, 'in point of philosophy, that the
inconvenience by gravitation of the blood should be irremediable. Why not erect
a bed higher than the operator's head, and lay the patient on it with the mouth
down, and the head a little projecting...? You will get sprinklings to be sure. But
take a fishing coat. And as for delicacy of operation, you would fare as well, in point
of position, as a painter doing angels on a cupola.'"

This was a brilliant suggestion which solved the problem of protection of the airway with absolute certainty — at the cost of some slight inconvenience to the surgeon. Because of this Miller rejected the idea at once and without making any attempt to solve the lighting difficulty by means of lamps, reflectors, mirrors, etc. He commented:

"No doubt. And this might do well enough in cases of polypus, for example, in which the operation is conducted by touch rather than by sight. But in excision of the jaw, and such like operations, a flood of light on the wounded part is indispensable in order to discern texture, and arrest haemorrhage; and the obtaining of this does not seem compatible with the peculiarity of the position ingeniously proposed."

Later on in his account Miller mentions another type of case in which, in his opinion, chloroform is contra-indicated.

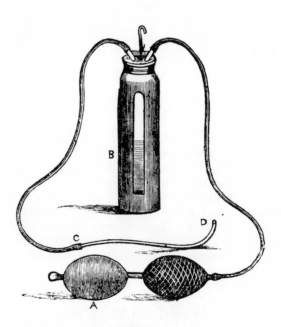

FIGURE 32

In *The Lancet* of December 14th, 1878, Joseph Mills, the administrator of chloroform at Bart's, described the use of this flexible mouth or nose tube for use with Junker's inhaler so that the anaesthetic could be administered during operations on the mouth and pharynx. Until he made this suggestion the chloroform was delivered into a facepiece which got in the surgeon's way.

"In the case of tracheotomy on account of a foreign body in the windpipe, anaesthesia must plainly be abstained from. It would facilitate instrumentation, no doubt; but at the transcendant risk of suffocation by unejected and accumulated blood."

Most of the early forms of vapourisers or insufflation bottles were designed as attempts to overcome the difficulties of access and to allow the administration of anaesthesia to be continued when the use of a facepiece was impossible; but they did not, in themselves, do anything to safeguard the airway from the entrance of blood or other material. The original Junker's apparatus[11] merely used a facepiece into which chloroform vapour was delivered by a hand-bulb and so was no better than any other mask from the point of view of easy access to the face. It was not until 1878 that Joseph Mills, of St. Bartholomew's Hospital in London, substituted, in place of the mask, a malleable metallic delivery tube through which the vapour was conveyed into the mouth or nose.[12] This invention was, at the time, an invaluable aid in the management of these awkward cases.

Gags and tongue depressors were introduced by the score, until their very names were legion. Again, their primary function was not protective for the larynx, but to make the field of operation reasonably accessible to both surgeon and anaesthetist. Mopping with sponges or the temporary placement of swabs and the like must have been the methods principally relied upon to preserve the airway.

Those who are, now, used to the calm and peaceful atmosphere of modern operations, in which the territories of the surgeon and the anaesthetist are usually controlled so that, even when they overlap, they are effectively protected by a cuffed intra-tracheal tube or some other device, will probably find it hard to imagine the difficulties that faced the anaesthetist of old in operations on the mouth and throat. Both surgeon and anaesthetist wanted access to the same cavity at the same time; the surgeon seemed to take an almost friendish delight in causing streams of blood to flow into the mouth and, no doubt, the anaesthetist always appeared to be in the way whenever the surgeon encountered any difficulty. A messy and gory business it was, and the patient easily and rapidly became too light and coughed a froth of blood and mucus into the surgeon's face and could easily be asphyxiated if the pool of blood in the mouth ran backwards, instead of forwards, or if the swabbing was not sufficiently rapid and efficient. All the time, both surgeon and anaesthetist were immersed in the pool of anaesthetic vapour which hung around the patient's face.

The problem of maintaining the airway in these difficult circumstances was mentioned by many people, a number of whom, thereafter, omitted to describe their own answers to it. Maurice H. Collis, who was Surgeon to the Meath Hospital and the County Dublin Infirmary, referred, in 1868, to cleft palate operations and said that he had used chloroform in all his cases during a period of two years and a half;[13] he gave no details whatsoever of the method of anaesthesia. F. Le Gros Clark, of St. Thomas' Hospital in London, advised caution and said:

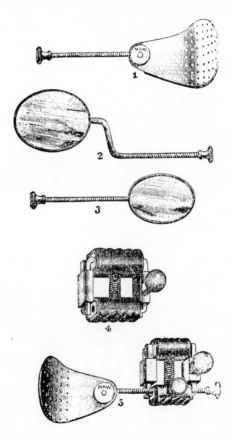

FIGURE 33

John Ward Cousins, a surgeon in Portsmouth invented this gag with a throat guard, and wrote about it in the *British Medical Journal* early in 1888. It was made by Maw and Thompson. Number 4 is the gag itself, which can be opened and closed when in position between the teeth; the steel dental surfaces are covered with rubber. The lower dental bar is perforated once to take the shaft on which is mounted either a throat guard or a mirror. It was used for dental and other intra-oral operations.

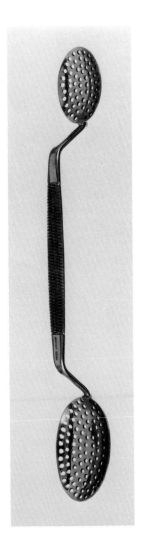

FIGURE 34
Carter Braine's oral spoons for protecting the airway during dental operations were introduced early in the 1900s. The gauze bowls of the earlier, and original model have been replaced by the much stronger perforated metal ones.

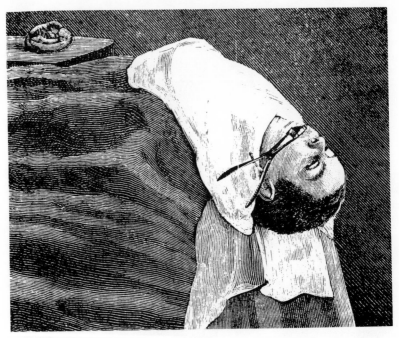

FIGURE 35

In the *British Medical Journal* of May 5th, 1894 James Murphy, of Sunderland, described this simple method of using gravity to prevent the entry of blood into the trachea during operations in the mouth and throat under general anaesthesia. He attributed the idea to Professeur Trélat, of La Charité Hospital in Paris.

"It is a dangerous practice to inhale chloroform in operations involving the interior of the mouth; although the risk is diminished if the sitting posture can be maintained. The intrusion of blood into the larynx, in any quantity, can scarcely fail to prove fatal under these circumstances; the admission of even a small quantity is sufficient to excite apprehension."[14]

One of the earliest gags to be fitted with a throat-guard was that of John Ward Cousins, a senior surgeon in Portsmouth, who may, possibly, have held at some time the world's record for the number of surgical gadgets he designed. The guard he described would not and could not be liquid-tight, but swabs could be placed up against it with the certainty of not losing them.[15] (I once lost a loose throat swab in the pharynx of a Russian prisoner-of-war in Germany. I got it out just in time, with a few seconds to spare. Those who have not committed this particular blunder will hardly believe how difficult it is to retrieve a blood-soaked and slippery swab which has gone well round the corner.) An alternative to Cousins' somewhat clumsy and fixed guard was Carter Braine's oral spoon which could be held in any desired position to catch blood and other debris. This apparatus was designed, particularly, for dental surgeons to use and was held by the anaesthetist immediately under the tooth being extracted.[16]

A very great, and simple, step forward in protecting the helpless larynx was reported in 1894 by James Murphy of Sunderland.[17] He admitted that it was not his own idea but that of Professeur Trélat of La Charité Hospital in Paris. This easy and effective method consisted, merely, of hanging the patient's head over the end of the operating table so that the mouth, nose and naso-pharynx were at a lower level than the larynx. Since the laws of gravity are rarely (if ever) suspended and liquids seldom (if ever) run uphill this was a most reliable dodge. At the time, and obvious as it seemed to be, it was probably the greatest French contribution to anaesthesia. It was, in effect, the method that was suggested in Edinburgh to Professor Miller by his inspired lay friend. Miller, as has been noted, turned the idea down without even trying it. Indeed, so little did he think of it that he did not even bother to record the name of its originator. Soon, complexities were added to this simple method and a special, low-fitting head-rest was described which could be clamped on to an ordinary kitchen table.[18] At that time (which was 1904) far more surgery was performed on the patient's kitchen table than now.

As surgeons grew bolder and more venturesome new methods had to be devised. The old ones were reckoned to be unreliable, inconvenient or both. The surgeon demanded absolute protection and, at the same time, wished to be able to put the patient's head in any position. Hahn and Trendelenburg

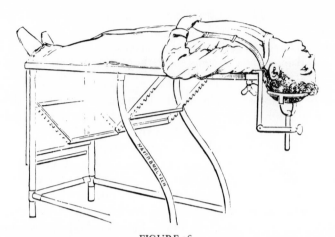

FIGURE 36

Dr. Frank Nyulasy, of Melbourne, described this head rest for intra-nasal operations in *The Lancet* on August 6th, 1904. It was made by Mayer and Meltzer, and was designed to clamp on to an ordinary kitchen table. It avoided the strained neck muscles which followed the use of the hanging head position and did away with the need for an assistant to hold the head steady during surgery.

introduced a new technique. They did a preliminary tracheostomy and inserted a tube which was surrounded, in the one case, by a sponge covering (Hahn's Tube) and in the other by an inflatable bag or cuff (Trendelenburg's Tampon).[19] These shut off the lungs and bronchi from the operative field, the head could be moved freely and, as an additional safeguard, the pharynx could be packed off if the site of the operation suggested that this might be helpful. An anaesthetic, vaporising device could then be firmly attached to the tracheostomy tube.

Others were content with a simple tracheostomy. Walter Cockle, who was anaesthetist to the Metropolitan Ear, Nose and Throat Hospital in London, described a small and simple apparatus for giving anaesthetics by this route.[20] He argued that "charging up a patient with chloroform", that is inducing deep anaesthesia and then stopping to allow the operation to proceed for a while during lightening, is dangerous and gives a wildly fluctuating and wholly unsatisfactory result; that a mask of any kind was cumbersome and got in the way of the surgeon, and that the flexible tube from a Junker's inhaler took up too much room when inserted into a tracheostomy tube. His little, square frame, mounted on the end of a fifteen inch long, malleable handle was intended to avoid these dangers.

A. E. Rockey, of Portland in Oregon was an improviser and put

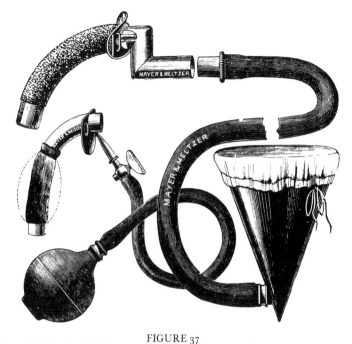

FIGURE 37

Dr. R. J. Probyn-Williams depicted these two types of apparatus, in 1901, for administering chloroform anaesthesia after a preliminary tracheostomy. The upper tube with the sponge seal is Hahn's tube; the lower one with an inflatable cuff is Trendelenburg's.

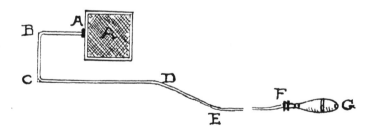

FIGURE 38

Walter Cockle's 1906 apparatus for maintaining anaesthesia through a tracheostomy consisted of a 1½ in. square frame fixed to a malleable handle and covered with a piece of lint on to which chloroform or A.C.E. was sprinkled. The handle could be bent to any convenient shape.

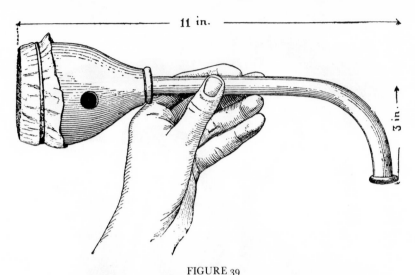

FIGURE 39

A. E. Rockey, of Portland, Oregon described this improvisation, in 1906, for the administration of anaesthesia during resection of the jaw. It was made from an old Hegar's ovarian trochar to which was attached an old Politzer bag with the top cut off and two holes made in its side. The top was covered with a fold of gauze, kept in place with a rubber band. The curved end was passed well into the throat after induction of anaesthesia, the tongue drawn forward with a stitch, and the mouth packed with gauze. This worked well in practice.

together an apparatus for intra-pharyngeal use out of bits and pieces of old surgical equipment.[21] This worked well and was a fore-runner of later airways fitted with inflatable rubber bags which, within their limits, worked well.

The very first airway I could trace, which was crude compared to its improved form, was designed by Frederic Hewitt who was, incidentally, Anaesthetist to His Majesty King Edward the Seventh and on the staff of both The London Hospital and St. George's Hospital, London. Introduced in 1908,[22] this was a straight rubber tube with a bite block; the shape of the tube was, probably, very soon changed to a moulded curve which conformed to the shape of the tongue and oro-pharynx. Strange to say, I could find no reference to this modification.

Many people, before (and even after) the adoption of intra-tracheal techniques, made use of airways and packings of various sorts. In 1904, P. Watson Williams used a pair of forceps with a double curve to place and hold a pack in the post-nasal space.[23] H. M. Page, anaesthetist to Guy's Hospital in London, used a pharyngeal pack and double naso-pharyngeal

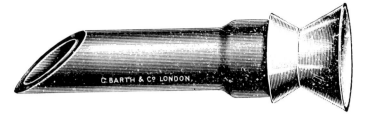

FIGURE 40
Hewitt's airway, with its original, straight, rubber tube.

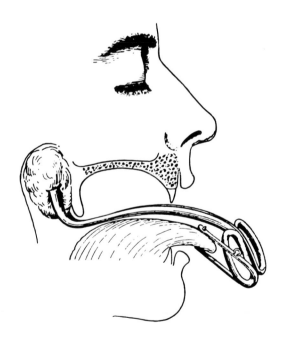

FIGURE 41
P. Watson Williams' post-nasal plug forceps also provided a means of pulling the tongue forward.

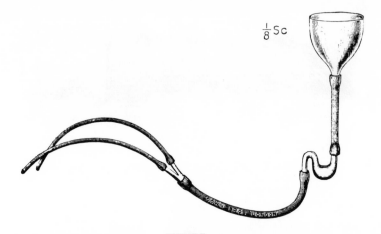

$\frac{1}{8}$ Sc

FIGURE 42

H. M. Page, anaesthestist to Guy's Hospital, London described these nasal tubes for the administration of ether during head and neck operations in *The Lancet* of August 7th, 1909. His idea was an adaptation of that originally by Crile. The nasal tubes were inserted until the distal ends were at the level of the epiglottis, and the pharynx was packed with gauze. An ether trap was provided.

tubes to protect the airway and administer anaesthesia.[24] Much later, in 1935, Sir Francis Shipway, also of Guy's Hospital, designed an ordinary, curved airway fitted with an inflatable cushion to act as a barrier between the nose and larynx during intranasal operations.[25] It had a side tube which enabled the anaesthetic to be continued during operations in the front of the mouth. Naturally, this was not effective in operations which were too far back. Leech produced an airway of similar form in Canada, but the pharyngeal blocker in his model was moulded from solid rubber instead of being inflatable.[26] Ideas such as these were still being put forward comparatively recently. In 1939, W. H. Marshall made use of a combined gas-delivery tube with a sponge pack attached to it,[27] and, in 1944, Dr. Rowbotham, then of the R.A.M.C., described the use of a separate, inflatable, rubber pharyngeal balloon which could be slipped on to a Magill's endotracheal tube and its position could be adjusted so that, when the tube lay properly in the larynx, the inflatable cuff was able to push the soft palate up against the posterior pharyngeal wall to isolate, and protect, the larynx during nasal operations.[28]

Dr. Franz Kuhn, of Kassel in Germany, described a simple and effective intra-tracheal tube in 1905, and this answered its purpose very well in all operations on the mouth or nose and gave perfect protection to the larynx

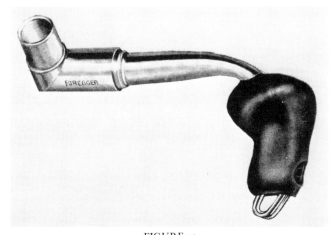

FIGURE 43

A Canadian airway, designed by Leech and made by Foregger, which had a solid rubber bulb moulded so that it would occlude the pharynx.

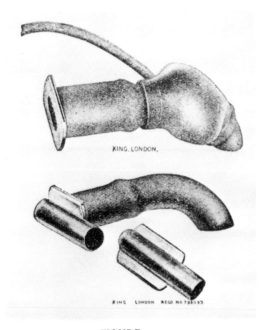

FIGURE 44

An English, occlusive airway designed by Sir Francis Shipway which had an inflatable cuff. It was designed for intra-nasal operations, and had a side-fitting tube through which the anaesthetic could be given without interfering with the surgeon.

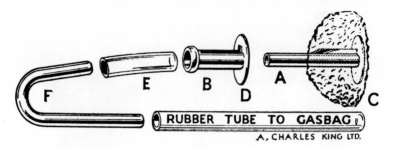

FIGURE 45

W. H. Marshall's combined gas-delivery tube and sponge pack. The sponge was held between the collar on A and that on B; the rubber tube, E, fitted over A and jammed B in position. After induction, the sponge which was dampened was pushed into the pharynx.

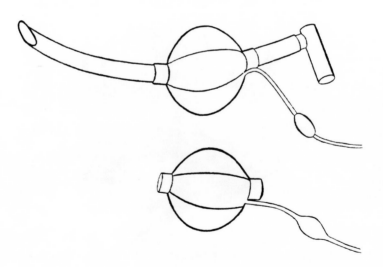

FIGURE 46

Rowbotham's inflatable pharyngeal cuff which was slipped on to a Magill's tube and blown up to occlude the pharynx, and to push the soft palate up against the posterior pharyngeal wall.

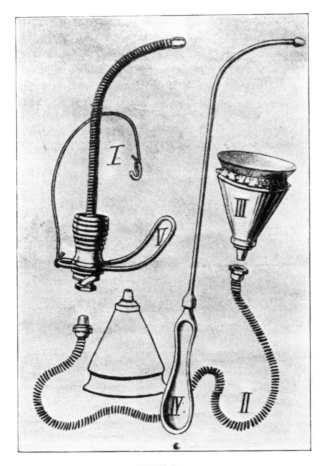

FIGURE 47

Kuhn's early instruments for tactile intubation of the larynx. I is the intra-tracheal tube to which a string, hook, and stout wire loop are attached for fixation although, in practice, the tube was kept in place by gauze packing in the pharynx, which protected the larynx. IV is the introducer on which the tube was threaded and III is the cone on to which ether or chloroform was poured.

provided that the gauze packing was inserted carefully.[29] I frequently used this tube to administer anaesthetics while I was a prisoner-of-war during the Second World War. It was simple and indestructible and, fortunately, did not need batteries since these were not available at the time.

(There will have to be a long parenthesis here, because there is a subject

109

to be discussed which does not properly fit into this chapter. On the other hand, I have no idea where else to put it. Anyway, it has to do with throat operations. In 1893 Mr. Dundas Grant, of the Central London Throat and Ear Hospital, stated that he had been using nitrous oxide (administered by his friend Mr. Sibley Read) to provide anaesthesia for the removal of tonsils and adenoids while avoiding the dangers associated with chloroform.[30] He wrote again just a fortnight later[31] in the happy and invulnerable position of one who can say "I told you so", because another death during tonsillectomy under chloroform anaesthesia had occurred on the very day that his first letter was published.

A few weeks later Mr. Wyatt Wingrave, an Assistant Surgeon and formerly Anaesthetist to the Central London Throat and Ear Hospital, wrote of his experience of removing tonsils and adenoids in 1100 cases, about ninety per cent of which received nitrous oxide alone, the remainder receiving gas supplemented by ether.[32] Only one patient, who recovered completely, caused him any concern whatsoever and this record he compared with five deaths during tonsillectomy performed under chloroform anaesthesia between May 1892 and August 1893. He concluded that, in the circumstances, nitrous oxide was practically harmless. Early in the following year, W. G. Holloway, who was at the time Registrar and Anaesthetist at the same hospital, reported that there had been two more deaths during adenoidectomies under chloroform within the previous fortnight.[33] He knew that, in one of the cases, the dangers of chloroform had been pointed out and the use of nitrous oxide recommended as a safe alternative, but without avail. He also added that, by now, nitrous oxide had been used at his hospital for two thousand such cases without accident. In the next two months, two more chloroform deaths were recorded — one at Bradford in a child with a hare-lip and cleft palate, and the other at Oxford in a child aged seven during adenoidectomy.[34] In both cases there was blood in the trachea and bronchi at necropsy.

In 1902, J. H. Chaldecott (who was then Anaesthetist at the Metropolitan Throat and Ear Hospital in London, and had earlier worked at the Central London Throat, Nose and Ear Hospital) pointed out that there had been more than 50 deaths reported during tonsil and adenoid operations which should, really, be virtually free from danger. Chaldecott said that the operation had been "perverted by the use of chloroform into one of the most immediately deadly in any of the long list of surgical operations". He also observed that many people said that tonsils and adenoids could not be satisfactorily dealt with under nitrous oxide or ether but replied to this criticism by pointing out that, at the Metropolitan and Central London

Throat Hospitals, some twenty thousand cases had been safely and properly operated upon in this way.[35]

In 1919 Frederick Sydenham, of Birmingham, attempted to sum up by saying that, after a large number of letters about the suitability of chloroform as an anaesthetic for tonsillectomy, there remained much conflict of opinion. His own view can be inferred from the fact that he had done sixteen thousand cases in twenty years — the first ten years with, and the second ten years *without anaesthesia*. Of his later method he wrote 'If it had been universally followed the fifty-six deaths recorded . . . would not have occurred."[36]

Perhaps not; but this seems to be where we came in. The wheel has turned full circle and is back where it started. James Syme removed the jaw without anaesthesia seventeen years after it was available; Frederick Sydenham removed tonsils in the twentieth century without anaesthesia, seventy-two years after it was available. *Plus ça change, plus c'est la même chose.* The simple alternative of securing good anaesthesia, apparently, never occurred to either of them. Would you like to have your tonsils taken out without an anaesthetic — however skilled the operator?)

Why the bracket? Perhaps you have forgotten. I told you a page or two back that it was a long parenthesis.

REFERENCES

[1] Bigelow, H. J. (1846) Insensibility during surgical operations produced by inhalation. *Boston Medical and Surgical Journal*, **35**, 309–317.

[2] Anonymous. (1847) Operations without pain. *Lancet*, **1**, 54.

[3] Warren, J. M. (1847) Inhalation of ether. *Boston Medical and Surgical Journal*, **36**, 149–162.

[4] Hayward, G. (1847) Some account of the first use of sulphuric ether by inhalation in surgical practice. *Boston Medical and Surgical Journal*, **36**, 229–234.

[5] Syme, J. (1865) Excision of the tongue. *Lancet*, **1**, 115.

[6] Anonymous. (1851) A mirror on the practice of Medicine and Surgery in the hospitals of London. *Lancet*, **1**, 545–546.

[7] Snow, J. (1858) *On chloroform and other anaesthetics.* London: Churchill.

[8] Leech, P. (1904) Cancer of Tongue. *Medical Annual*, 688–695.

[9] Turner, A. L. (1937) *Story of a great hospital — The Royal Infirmary of Edinburgh 1729–1929.* Edinburgh: Oliver and Boyd.

[10] Miller, J. (1850) *The principles of surgery.* Edinburgh: Black.

[11] Junker, F. E. (1867) Description of a new apparatus for administering narcotic vapours. *Medical Times and Gazette*, **2**, 590.

[12] Mills, J. (1878) On a method of administering chloroform for operations about the mouth. *Lancet*, **2**, 839.

[13] Collis, M. H. (1868) Chloroform in cleft palate. *British Medical Journal*, **1**, 131.

[14] Clark, F. Le G. (1869) Lesions of the neck and throat. *British Medical Journal*, **2**, 203–206.

[15] Cousins, J. W. (1888) New gag with throat guard. *British Medical Journal*, **1**, 360–361.

[16] Anonymous. (1925) *Catalogue of the Dental Manufacturing Company*, 21.

[17] Murphy, J. (1894) A simple means of preventing the entrance of blood into the trachea during operations about the mouth. *British Medical Journal*, **1**, 964–965.

[18] Nyulasy, F. A. (1904) A head-rest for post-nasal operations. *Lancet*, **2**, 381.

[19] Probyn-Williams, R. J. (1901) *A practical guide to the administration of anaesthetics*. London: Longmans, Green and Co.

[20] Cockle, W. P. (1906) A new method of administering an anaesthetic through a tracheostomy tube. *Lancet*, **2**, 717–718.

[21] Rockey, A. E. (1906) A device for anaesthesia in resection of the jaw. *Medical Record*, **69**, 906.

[22] Hewitt, F. W. (1908) An artificial "air-way" for use during anaesthetisation. *Lancet*, **1**, 490–491.

[23] Williams, P. W. (1908) Plugging the posterior nares. *Medical Annual*, 398–399.

[24] Page, H. M. (1909) A method of giving ether by means of nasal tubes. *Lancet*, **2**, 364.

[25] Shipway, Sir F. (1935) Airway for intranasal operations. *British Medical Journal*, **1**, 767.

[26] Clement, F. W. (1951) *Nitrous oxide–oxygen anaesthesia*. 3rd Ed. Philadelphia: Lea and Febiger.

[27] Marshall, W. H. (1939) Combined sponge and gas-delivery tube. *Lancet*, **2**, 692.

[28] Rowbotham, E. S. (1944) An inflatable pharyngeal tube. *Lancet*, **2**, 15–16.

[29] Kuhn, F. (1905) Die perorale Intubation mit und ohne Druck. *Deutsche Zeitschrift für Chirurgie*, **78**, 467–520.

[30] Grant, D. (1893) Deaths under anaesthetics. *Lancet*, **2**, 343.

[31] Grant, D. Nitrous oxide anaesthesia for the removal of tonsils and adenoids. *Lancet*, **2**, 443–444.

[32] Wingrave, W. (1893) Anaesthesia for operations on the throat and nose. *British Medical Journal*, **2**, 707–708.

[33] Holloway, W. G. (1894) Chloroform in nasal growths. *Lancet*, **1**, 64.

[34] Anonymous. (1894) Deaths under chloroform. *British Medical Journal* **1**, 649.

[35] Chaldecott, J. H. (1902) The choice of an anaesthetic for short operations upon the throat and nose. *Lancet*, 743–744.

[36] Sydenham, F. (1919) Enucleation of tonsils without an anaesthetic. *British Medical Journal*, **2**, 151–152.

CHAPTER 9

HOW STOOD HOSPITAL PROGRESS IN 1883?
A HOSPITAL ENQUIRY

"Those who urge the general employment of dangerous remedies on the plea that, in their own hands, they have hitherto proved safe, remind us of the quibble of the Scotch judge, who had never, he asserted, known any one die of drinking, though he had, he acknowledged, known many lost while learning the art."

— EDITORIAL, *British Medical Journal,* (1869) **2**, 589.

In 1882, a year in which disquiet and uncertainty about the safety of chloroform was being voiced, *The Lancet* noted that the managers of the Royal Infirmary in Glasgow had proposed to lay down rules for the guidance of their surgeons in the administration of anaesthetics.[1] On reflection, however, it was thought that the natural reluctance of the surgeons there to receive instructions in the subject from a lay body meant that the matter could be more easily dealt with by the Infirmary's medical committee.

The committee, thus set up, then made enquiries about the administration of anaesthetics, especially chloroform, in various large hospitals. A nine point questionnaire was sent out by the committee; how many hospitals were sent this we are not told, but replies were received from the following twenty hospitals.

> Newcastle upon Tyne Infirmary
> Glasgow Western Infirmary
> Perth Infirmary
> Edinburgh Royal Infirmary
> Dundee Royal Infirmary
> Aberdeen Royal Infirmary
> Greenock Royal Infirmary
> Dumfries Royal Infirmary
> Manchester Royal Infirmary
> Liverpool Royal Infirmary
> Bristol Royal Infirmary
> Sheffield Royal Infirmary
> St. Thomas' Hospital, London
> Guy's Hospital, London
> Westminster Hospital, London
> King's College Hospital, London

University College Hospital, London
St. Mary's Hospital, London
Leeds General Infirmary
St. Vincent's Hospital, Dublin

So replies were received from twenty hospitals, seven Scottish, one Irish and twelve English, the latter being equally divided between London and the provinces. In May 1883, *The Lancet* printed a summary of the Glasgow committee's findings.[2] One of the points raised in the questionnaire had been statistical, relating to the number of beds, etc. in the hospitals and was referred to in passing; the replies to the other eight questions were discussed in some detail.

Question 1. "Are there any formal regulations issued with the sanction of the directors of your hospital with respect to the use and administration of anaesthetics, especially chloroform?"

Most of the hospitals replied that they had no regulations whatsoever, but there were seven exceptions to this general pattern. Aberdeen had a "regular chloroformist for all staff operations", and at St. Thomas' there were two anaesthetists — a senior and a junior — with complete sets of rules for their guidance. At King's College Hospital there was a special administrator and, at St. Mary's Hospital, it seemed that the medical administrator acted as the anaesthetist. At Leeds the house physician did this work by himself when the need arose; more junior doctors were allowed to give anaesthetics only if their senior colleagues were present. This practice also seems to have been followed at Newcastle and at St. Vincent's Hospital, Dublin.

Question 2. "Is there any special instruction given in the hospital, or in the medical school, on the above subject?"

At the Glasgow Western and in Dundee, Perth, Greenock, Dumfries, Bristol and Sheffield there was no special tuition. Instruction "in some form or other" was given at the other hospitals.

Question 3. "Are the resident medical and surgical officers permitted to administer chloroform without the presence of the visiting surgeon, or other member of the senior staff of the hospital? And, if so, under what restrictions, if any?"

The Lancet considered this to be an important point, but its account of the committee's conclusions is ambiguous.

"On this important point we learn that in *none* of the hospitals named, except St. Vincent's and Dundee, are there restrictions placed on the resident surgeons in the giving of chloroform. In Glasgow Western it is required that two residents shall be present. In Dundee there is but one house-surgeon, and he administers only in the presence of the superintendent or one of the staff. At St. Thomas's, the 'qualified resident officers' administer anaesthetics without the visiting surgeons: at Guy's the residents may do so in the absence of their seniors, 'when absolutely necessary;' in Westminster, they may do so 'when occasion may arise — e.g., for the performance of some minor surgical operation, the reduction of a dislocated limb,' &c.: in King's College, they do so 'in emergencies.'"

Question 4. "Are such resident medical officers assistant or principal officers?"

Almost always the residents who gave anaesthetics were assistants, and not principals. At University College Hospital they were principals. In some of the hospitals there were two classes of residents, the house-physicians or surgeons who were qualified, and their assistants who were not.

Question 5. "Are such resident medical officers, in every instance, men legally qualified to practise medicine and surgery? And for what period have they practised or been qualified to practise? Or has any special instruction in the use of anaesthetics been required of them as a qualification for their appointment?"

Most of the hospitals which responded to the questionnaire required their residents to be medically qualified. University College Hospital, Leeds General Infirmary and Dumfries Royal Infirmary, however, did not.

As a rule, the residents were recently qualified doctors. In only five of the hospitals was instruction in anaesthesia thought to be important for the residents and in the remaining fifteen it was not felt necessary that any of these men should be instructed in anaesthetics before administering them.

Question 6. "Is it permitted to assistants not legally qualified in surgical wards to administer chloroform or other anaesthetics? and, if so, under what restrictions, if any?"

Most of the hospitals did not allow unqualified men to administer anaesthetics. However, in certain circumstances (usually the supervising presence of a senior colleague), they were allowed to do so at Aberdeen, Newcastle, Liverpool and Bristol. At University College Hospital in London chloroform was given by unqualified men "without supervision". To the astonishment of *The Lancet* the matron at Perth Infirmary frequently gave chloroform under the supervision of a medical officer.

Question 7. "Is there any specialist appointed for the administration of anaesthetics?"

Only four of the twenty hospitals had specialist chloroformists — Aberdeen, St. Thomas', Guy's and King's College.

Question 8. "Have fatal accidents occurred in your hospital during the medical or surgical administration of chloroform? and, if so, has the occurrence of such accidents led to any practical (even if not formal) restrictions as regards its administration, as aforesaid?"

Six of the hospitals claimed complete immunity from such accidents. These were at Perth, Dundee, Aberdeen, Leeds Infirmary, King's College and St. Vincent's where, it was stated categorically, that no deaths from chloroform had occurred. I have definite evidence that this claim was not true as far as two of these hospitals were concerned — Leeds and Aberdeen; and my records are not, by any means, complete.

In 1871 there was a case report from the Royal Infirmary in Aberdeen of a 37-year-old man who died under chloroform anaesthesia following the first incision of an operation for hernia.[3] Three years later, at the Leeds General Infirmary, a man of 48 died under chloroform just after the operation for amputation of a finger had begun.[4]

An anonymous gentleman, who aptly chose the pseudonym "Scrutator", noticed the mistaken claim about Aberdeen made in the committee's report. He promptly wrote to the editor, and his letter was published the following week.[5]

"In *The Lancet* of to-day, in the article on the administration of anaesthetics in hospitals, I see that, in answer to Question 8 of the Committee appointed by the Glasgow Infirmary, it is stated that no deaths from chloroform have occurred at, among others, the Aberdeen Infirmary. I distinctly remember being present on one occasion in the operating theatre there, when the late Professor Pirrie was about to perform Wood's operation for the radical cure of hernia, and when the patient died on the table during the administration of an anaesthetic, and before the operation had commenced. . . . I have always believed that the anaesthetic used was chloroform, but of this I cannot speak with certainty. . . . As it is, I have thought it worth while to record the fact of the death. In statistics, above all things, the first requisite is accuracy."

How right "Scrutator" was — about the desirability, indeed the absolute necessity, of accuracy.

The Glasgow Infirmary's investigating committee said that the other hospitals admitted that deaths had occurred "and will occur from time to time" but, with the exception of St. Mary's Hospital, no practical changes were made following these fatalities. The Glasgow Western Infirmary reported that there had been two chloroform deaths during the previous eight and a half years, and in both cases one or more of the visiting surgeons had been present. The Liverpool Royal Infirmary admitted two deaths in five years, one from chloroform and one from ether. Dumfries reported one — "on that occasion the whole resident and visiting staff were present." In Guy's Hospital, the deaths from anaesthesia amounted to one or two a year.

The numbers of deaths which occurred at the other hospitals are not mentioned. I have records of some which happened in Edinburgh.

In 1853, Dr. Dunsmore had a death at the Royal Infirmary during an operation for urethral stricture.[6] Dr. Gillespie, senior surgeon to the Royal Infirmary, and President of the Royal College of Surgeons of Edinburgh met another in 1871 during the reduction of a dislocated shoulder.[7] Dr. Gillespie added "it is the first fatal case which has occurred to myself as hospital surgeon during the last fifteen years".[8] The editor of the journal noted that the immunity from fatal results at Edinburgh had been "remarkably prolonged" and noticed the careful, and rather artificial, phrasing used by Gillespie — "myself as hospital surgeon" — and pressed the matter, whereupon the surgeon admitted that he had also had a death from chloroform in his private practice.[9] One would think far more highly of those who told the whole truth openly, willingly and honestly, rather than waiting for it to be prised out of them by others. Nothing further was said about the Editor's belief that there had been, by then, four or five deaths from chloroform in the wards of the Royal Infirmary.

Later, in 1880, James Spence, then Professor of Surgery in Edinburgh, said that only seven or eight deaths during chloroform had occurred at the Royal Infirmary during the previous thirty-two years.[10] Shortly after Spence's statement another death occurred in his hospital under chloroform.[11] So that made eight or nine fatal cases.

For most of the thirty-two years referred to by Professor Spence the average number of operations would be about three hundred a year, or a total of 9,600. (The rapid increase in the number of operations due to antiseptics did not really begin until after 1880.) Taking the more favourable figure of eight deaths at Edinburgh, rather than nine, this gives a death rate of about 1 in 1,200. This figure is not very different from many other series collected in various places. Careful records were kept at St. Bartholomew's Hospital in London and revealed a death rate from chloroform in that hospital of 1 in 1,236.[12] This point would scarcely be worth pointing out had not Edinburgh-trained people, from the time of Syme onwards, been so fond of pointing out their own fancied superiority in giving chloroform.

I cannot be certain what was in the Glaswegians' minds when they designed their questionnaire, but most of their questions seem to be more concerned with the calibre of the administrator than anything else. Not much comment was made about whether chloroform was inherently safe or not. However, the general impression left by the report is that anaesthesia, at that time, was an unorganised chaos, with no real attempts to ensure either efficiency or safety. This condemnation does not apply to any particular place, for there was very little to choose between any of the twenty hospitals who answered the questionnaire. Standards of anaesthesia in hospitals not involved in the report from Glasgow probably varied widely and in some, were better and, in others, worse than the examples quoted. In all probability, however, the average standard of anaesthetic practice can be deduced fairly accurately.

The final result of the investigation was that the committee of the Glasgow Royal Infirmary felt able to make certain recommendations. These the committee sent to "forty of the principal hospitals . . . from upwards of twenty of which they received detailed replies".[13] The recommendations were, firstly, that all new assistants should be instructed by the surgeons in the use of anaesthetics. Secondly, that preference should be given to assistants who had received tuition in anaesthesia. Thirdly, that surgeons should give certificates of competency when they were satisfied that their assistants knew about the techniques of administration of anaesthesia, their complications and the management of these. Fourthly, that assistants who gave anaesthetics must be legally qualified and should only administer anaesthesia in the absence of their seniors if they possessed a certificate of competency. Two further recommendations made provision for cases of extreme urgency, and the last were that careful records of all anaesthetics given in the surgeon's absence should be made and that, when a death occurred with an anaesthetic it must be reported to the hospital's committee.

With the benefit of hindsight it is obvious that the committee overlooked several factors which were important to its enquiry. At any rate, they made an attempt to find out why things were not going all that well, and to improve matters. So the questionnaire was not entirely wasted.

REFERENCES

[1] Anonymous. (1882) Glasgow. *Lancet*, **2**, 726.
[2] Anonymous. (1883) Administration of anaesthetics in hospitals. *Lancet*, **1**, 837–838.
[3] Anonymous. (1871) Death of a patient while under the influence of chloroform. *British Medical Journal*, **2**, 124.
[4] Anonymous. (1874) Death from chloroform. *British Medical Journal*, **2**, 141–142.
[5] Scrutator. (1883) Anaesthetics in hospitals. *Lancet*, **1**, 892.
[6] Anonymous. (1853) Deaths from chloroform. *British Medical Journal*, **2**, 971–972.
[7] Anonymous. (1871) Death from chloroform in the Edinburgh Royal Infirmary. *British Medical Journal*, **1**, 259.
[8] Anonymous. (1871) Death from chloroform in the Edinburgh Royal Infirmary. *British Medical Journal*, **1**, 288–289.
[9] Editorial. (1871) Deaths from anaesthetics. *British Medical Journal*, **1**, 480.
[10] Spence, J. (1880) Lecture introductory to the course on surgery. *Lancet*, **1**, 1–3.
[11] Anonymous. (1880) Death from chloroform. *British Medical Journal*, **1**, 178.
[12] Williams, W. R. (1890) The relative safety of anaesthetics. *Lancet*, **1**, 317.
[13] Anonymous. (1883) The Royal Infirmary, Glasgow. *Medical Times and Gazette*, **1**, 532–533.

CHAPTER 10

ANAESTHETICS BY A VERY GREAT SURGEON: SCHIZOPHRENIA IN EXCELSIS

In a once-famous, Victorian textbook of surgery there is a chapter on anaesthetics. It was written in three instalments, at different dates, and all three were printed together in the 1883 edition.[1]

When the first part of this chapter was written, in 1861, the author was what is conventionally called "an eminent surgeon"; that is, he was the Professor of Surgery at Glasgow University. Like all his colleagues of the time he was an artisan with a knowledge of anatomy — a mechanic whose dirty methods frustrated most of his work and limited it within very narrow boundaries. Except for the fact that he and his contemporaries had made use of the advantages of anaesthesia for some years their surgery differed little from that of the old barber-surgeons. It was slightly less hurried, because the patient was no longer conscious during their surgery, but it was almost as dangerous and crude, when judged by our present day standards. At the time, the author was no more and no less eminent than his contemporaries.

The second instalment, dating from 1870, was written in the year that James Syme had died and, by which time, the author of the chapter had succeeded him as Clinical Professor of Surgery at Edinburgh. By this time he had become someone more than "an eminent surgeon" since, before he had left Glasgow he had begun to revolutionise the whole of surgery by his work on antisepsis during operations.

The first steps had been halting and uncertain, and had met with a great deal of opposition. The older surgeons were satisfied with the thirty per cent mortality which followed their operations and could not visualise any possibility of improvement. They, therefore, saw no reason at all why they should not merely strop their knives and, straightway, plunge them into their patients. On the Continent, however, the Professor had acquired a great reputation — long before he acquired his full stature in his own country. By 1882, when he wrote the third instalment, he had again changed his job and had become Professor of Clinical Surgery at King's College in London. Opposition to his opinions was, by then, dying down because the results of his new practice spoke for themselves. The revolution which he had initiated was in full swing, and parts of the body, hitherto barred to the surgeons, had become accessible. It was the beginning of abdominal surgery, the beginning of thoracic surgery and the beginning of neurosurgery.

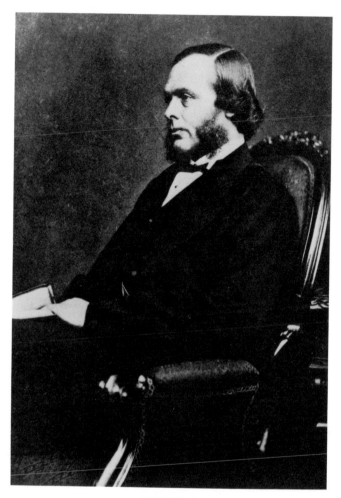

FIGURE 48

Joseph Lister, c. 1867.

Whitehall, December 26, 1883.

THE Queen has been pleased to direct Letters Patent to be passed under the Great Seal of the United Kingdom of Great Britain and Ireland, granting the dignity of a Baronet of the said United Kingdom unto Joseph Lister, of Park-crescent, in the parish of St. Marylebone, in the county of Middlesex, Esq., one of the Surgeons Extraordinary to Her Majesty, and the heirs male of his body lawfully begotten.

FIGURE 49
The announcement of Lister's baronetcy in the *London Gazette*.

Whitehall, February 8, 1897.

THE Queen has been pleased to direct Letters Patent to be passed under the Great Seal of the United Kingdom of Great Britain and Ireland, granting the dignity of a Baron of the said United Kingdom unto Sir Joseph Lister, Bart., President of the Royal Society, and the heirs male of his body lawfully begotten, by the name, style, and title of Baron Lister, of Lyme Regis, in the county of Dorset.

FIGURE 50
The announcement of Lister's barony in the *London Gazette*.

This revolution was due to one man, who stood out far above each and every one of his contemporary colleagues as a scientist and as an investigator.

He did not gain his position of unchallenged pre-eminence by making piddling, little improvements to individual operations, or by knocking a second or two off the time needed to perform an amputation. Instead, he completely remodelled the whole of operative surgery and changed it from a crude and dangerous handicraft into an expanding and much safer science. The Professor's name, of course, was Joseph Lister. He was born at Upton, in Essex, on 5th April, 1827 and had qualified from University College, London in 1852. He became a Baronet in 1883, and was created a Baron in 1897. He died, in his eighty-fifth year, on 10th February, 1912.

(For American, and other readers who know even less about the British "honours system" than I do, this is a rough idea of it.

If a person attains eminence in science, literature, local politics or whatever, he may be made a knight, which means that he is entitled to be called "Sir" and his wife "Lady". But this does not affect his family and the title dies when he dies. The next step upwards is a Baronetcy and this is similar to a knighthood but the title, when the holder dies, is passed on to the oldest son. This rank was, originally, invented by one of the Stuart kings as a method of raising money. It was sold, I think, for a sum of ten thousand pounds. Neither of these ranks entitle the possessor to sit in the House of Lords, which is the upper chamber of the English Parliament. The next step, however, does, and this is the rank of Baron. This title, and all above it, are hereditary titles. A barony is the lowest rank in the House of Lords; no medical man has, yet, risen above this rank, not even Lord Lister. The next step up is a Viscount, which title is out-ranked by an Earl. Then comes a Marquess, and, last but not least, right at the top is a Duke.

Successful politicians, unsuccessful ones who must be got out of the House of Commons at all costs, brewers and newspaper owners tend to be promoted to the lowest of these various degrees, but, even so, it is essential to brew a lot of beer or to own a lot of newspapers because these distinctions are not given to the smaller fry. The quality of the beer or the papers is not reckoned to be important. The highest rank, of Duke, is strictly reserved for those who have, often, done little apart from having chosen their parents carefully. Dukedoms have been created very rarely in recent times and the only way, by and large, to become one is to choose one of the existing dukes as a father. Becoming a duke used to have many advantages; it usually carried with it great wealth, from the ownership of land, and magnificent and enormous residences inherited from ancestors. Nowadays, crushing taxation on large incomes and death duties, or whatever, which range up to an enormous percentage, have reduced both income and capital accumulation to such an extent that stately homes can only be kept going by throwing them open to the public as show places at so many pence a head. Many of the stately homes do this — they have to — to keep going at all.

There can be no question about it, Lister was the greatest surgeon who ever lived. He was most definitely not, however, the greatest surgical technician who ever lived and, why he was asked to write about anaesthesia is beyond all comprehension. Joseph Clover should have written these particular articles instead of Lister. Nonetheless, Lister's remarks are worth examining, especially if their shortcomings are considered. He extolled the benefits of chloroform uncritically.

"Such being the great benefits conferred by this agent, it is melancholy to reflect that in many parts of Europe, and even of the United Kingdom, it is either withheld altogether or given so scantily as to be nearly useless. This arises from fear, inspired by several fatal cases that have occurred. But when I state that Mr. Syme has given chloroform about five thousand times without ever meeting a death, and that Sir J. Simpson's experience, also very extensive, has, so far as I am aware, been equally satisfactory, it is clear that it may be used so as to be practically free from any risk whatever."

This statement is simply not true as far as Simpson was concerned. As I pointed out in another essay[2] Simpson encountered a death from chloroform in 1855, which was six years before this part of Lister's article was written. In 1870 he reported a chloroform death on the table during one of his own operations.

Nowhere in these writings does Lister give any figures about his own cases and how they fared under chloroform.

"How then are the fatal cases to be accounted for? Heart disease has been supposed to be a common cause of them; and it is a prevalent opinion that it is highly dangerous to administer chloroform to persons affected with cardiac disorder.
"It happens that the only death I ever witnessed under chloroform occurred in a person whose heart proved, on examination, to be extensively affected with fatty degeneration, such as would be regarded as sufficient explanation of sudden death under any circumstances."

Lister then goes on to say that the patient was very lightly anaesthetised and died, suddenly, on the first incision. Hannah Greener[2] and hundreds of other, often young, healthy people died in a similar way. Had they all got diseased hearts? It seems unlikely.

"From these facts we can hardly doubt that death was a consequence of the shock of the operation acting on a diseased heart; and the only question is whether the circumstance that he had taken chloroform promoted that result ... such a thing seems altogether improbable, as we have seen that chloroform protects the heart from the effects of shock. My own impression is that if it had been pushed to the usual degree the fatal occurrence would have been averted."

Lister had previously mentioned a case of double amputation at the hip and shoulder joints after a railway accident, in which the moribund patient lived longer than was expected following an operation "performed as a forlorn hope" under chloroform. On this evidence he based his opinion that chloroform prevented shock. He admitted, however, that overdose with chloroform was possible, and that he had, himself, accidentally killed a laboratory animal in this way during an experiment. This occurred in 1853. Lister had been asked to anaesthetise a donkey for some experiment on its heart and so had chloroformed the animal and then maintained artificial respiration with a large bellows connected with a tube tied into the animal's windpipe. The chest was opened and, later, the animal began to come round.

"To avert this I removed the bellows, and poured into them a considerable quantity of chloroform, and resumed the artificial respiration with energy for a short time, the natural respiratory movements meanwhile continuing; when suddenly the heart, which lay exposed before us ceased to beat ..."

He then mentioned John Snow's accurate inhaler for chloroform which had been used by its inventor in more than four thousand cases with only one fatality which, in all probability, had not been due to the chloroform. Snow considered that when chloroform was given from a folded towel the concentration of the vapour varied uncontrollably and often led to overdosage. Lister, however, was not impressed by the argument.

"But the cloth being the means which has been used from the first in Edinburgh, with success even superior to Dr. Snow's, I have been long satisfied that his argument was fallacious; yet as his special devotion to the subject, and the valuable facts which he has communicated regarding it, render his opinion influential, I have thought it worth while to subject a matter of such great practical importance to experimental inquiry; and, about the usual quantity of liquid being employed, I find that, so far from the amount of chloroform given off from the cloth being in dangerous proportion to the air inhaled, the whole quantity which evaporates from the under surface, even when the rate is most rapid, *viz.* just after the liquid has been poured upon it, is below Dr. Snow's limit of perfect security against primary failure of the heart."

Lister inferred that, with rare exceptions due to idiosyncrasy, most fatalities were caused by overdosage. He pointed out that most of them were demonstrably not in severe or formidable operations but had occurred in relatively trivial ones. Had he taken the trouble to read the various, published reports he would have realised that most of the unfortunate patients were quite definitely not overdosed — they were not even properly under. He then went on, with that self-confidence which can be acquired by total ignorance of the subject, to explain this fictitious overdosage.

"The only rational explanation of this seems to be, that when some great operation is to be performed, like the amputation of a thigh or the removal of a stone from the bladder, plenty of well-qualified assistants are present, and each of them, including the giver of chloroform, is duly impressed with the importance of his office, and bestows the requisite pains upon it. But when some trifle is to be done, the whole affair is apt to be regarded too lightly, and the administration of the anaesthetic is perhaps confided to some unsuitable person, who also allows his attention to be distracted by other matters."

This is plausible, very plausible; but it bears no relation to the facts, and it is in flat contradiction to Lister's own practice. He, like many other eminent surgeons, had his anaesthetics given by unsupervised medical students in all cases, even the major ones. That is, by the very unsuitable persons referred to above. Later in his article, Lister says that: "The notion that extensive experience is required for the administration of chloroform is quite erroneous . . ." How then, one is entitled to ask, can anybody be "unsuitable" to give it?

Lister recorded his opinion, borrowed from his father-in-law Professor Syme, that concern with the pulse during chloroform anaesthesia was a mistake, and that any preliminary examination of the patient was dangerous.

"The very prevalent opinion that the pulse is the most important symptom in the administration of chloroform is certainly a most serious mistake. As a general rule, the safety of the patient will be most promoted by disregarding it altogether, so that the attention may be devoted exclusively to the breathing . . . preliminary examination of the chest, often considered indispensable, is quite unnecessary, and more likely to induce the dreaded syncope, by alarming the patient, than to avert it."

He also repeated Syme's maxim that "every case for operation is a case for chloroform". It is quite fair to conclude that Lister's attitude to anaesthesia was "Be as careless as you like; don't examine the patient beforehand; don't observe him overmuch during anaesthesia; allow anybody to give the anaesthetic, whether he knows anything about it or not; no training, no skill and no experience is needed. Don't take any precautions of any sort whatsoever."

"Chloroform is universally applicable in the various departments of surgery, except in some few cases in which the assistance of the patient is required, and in operations involving copious haemorrhage into the mouth. Blood may trickle in small amount into the pharynx without risk of choking, deglutition being carried on unconsciously during anaesthesia."

Altogether, Lister was a curious and inexplicable paradox. A few years after he wrote the account of anaesthesia he was to become the greatest iconoclast and reformer in the history of medicine since William Harvey, some three centuries before. But he was a dyed-in-the-wool, diehard obstructionist in one particular aspect of it — anaesthesia. He advocated just one careless method, with no possibility of improvement considered or desired, with no thought of progress of any kind, then or in the future. How could there be any progress with anaesthesia allocated wholly to students and thought of as a subject for which experience was not necessary?

I can understand men who are resistant to new ideas, and who are antagonistic to progress, even if I do not always sympathise with them. I can, also, understand men who are always looking for something new, or something better. But, to find both characteristics highly developed in one and the same person is beyond me altogether. To me, the combination just does not make sense.

The second part of Lister's account of anaesthesia was written in 1870. *Part One*, his earlier article, was published unchanged. *Part Two* began:

"The nine years which have passed since the above article was written have tended to confirm its main doctrines. . . . Mr. Syme, though he continued to within the last two years in the full activity of his career as an operator, never lost a patient through its use, either in public or private practice. Further, I believe I am correct in stating that no case of death from chloroform has occurred during these nine years, in the operating theatre of either the Edinburgh or the Glasgow Infirmary, two of the largest hospitals in Great Britain."

Superficially, this seems to be an impressive account; but notice the careful wording, that no deaths had occurred *"in the operating theatre"*. Chloroform deaths had happened in the wards of both the Edinburgh and the Glasgow Infirmary. In addition, we should remember the small number of operations performed at the time. Before Lister's antisepsis enlarged the scope of surgery the average number of operations performed each year in a large hospital was about 300, or some 2,700 in the nine years to which

Lister referred. The Registrar-General's figures show that, in 1870, there were 14 deaths from chloroform anaesthesia, and that was just in England and Wales. The case for Lister's defence of chloroform was not nearly so convincing as it sounded. Nonetheless, he continued unabashed.

"Yet in both these institutions a folded towel on which the anaesthetic liquid is poured, unmeasured and unstinted, is still the only apparatus employed in the administration: preliminary examination of the heart is never thought of, and during the inhalation the pulse is entirely disregarded; but vigilant attention is kept upon the respiration, and in the case of its obstruction, firm traction upon the tongue is promptly resorted to."

Lister believed that firm traction on the tongue, often with artery forceps, acted not only mechanically but also by some mechanism which worked on the nervous system.

He still maintained that no particular skill was necessary for the administration of chloroform, and that the appointment of a special administrator of chloroform to a hospital was not only unnecessary, but also had "the great disadvantage of investing the administration of chloroform with an air of needless mystery". The views he put forward on "idiosyncrasy" to chloroform were, characteristically, didactic.

"... no one can say it is impossible that here and there an individual may be found so constituted that, without any undue proportion of the narcotic vapour to the air inhaled, the cardiac ganglia may fail before respiration is interfered with. But while freely admitting that such a thing is possible, I must repeat my firm conviction that this kind of idiosyncrasy is certainly 'so rare that it may practically be left out of consideration altogether'.... death from chloroform is almost invariably due to faulty administration."

And yet, Lister maintained, there was no need to make any effort to secure good administration! Care was not necessary, selection of patients pointless, skill not wanted, experience superfluous and training not required. He did admit, however, that the giving of chloroform was "better performed after some practical initiation".

The second article concluded with a few, casual remarks about other anaesthetic agents, about which Lister apparently knew even less than he did about chloroform. He scorned the North American claims that ether was far safer than chloroform, and attributed the Bostonians' indignation to envy or wounded pride. He did admit, though, that ether was useful for cases of ovariotomy, and others when post-anaesthetic vomiting was better avoided. As for ether's alleged safety, "the case may probably be fairly stated by saying that ether, being less potent, is less liable to cause death from mismanagement". He was similarly dismissive about nitrous oxide but did add that "for avoiding the brief but acute agony of tooth-extraction, it appears to be an unquestionable boon to humanity". Local anaesthesia produced by cold, Lister considered, had a useful though limited place in surgical practice.

Part Three was written, twelve years later, in 1882 and appeared, preceded by the two earlier and unaltered instalments. Lister was, clearly, not prepared to be critical of his earlier views or to recant, even though in the twelve year interval ether had largely superseded chloroform because of what he described as "its supposed greater safety".

Lister noted that ether was, at the time, given from special inhalers, such as those designed by Ormsby or Clover, the use of which involved some degree of asphyxia. This, he said, produced many dangers which did not arise when chloroform was administered in the manner which he had previously described.

"The experience of the past twelve years has confirmed me in the soundness of this doctrine; and I venture to think it not undeserving of careful consideration, that in my hospital cases I have still entrusted the administration of the chloroform, not to a specialist or to a person of very large experience, but to a succession of senior students, changing from month to month, whose only qualification for the duty is that they must previously have served the office of dresser, and that they strictly carry out certain simple instructions, among which is that of never touching the pulse, in order that their attention may not be distracted from the respiration. I have also systematically abstained from making any preliminary examination of the heart, thus avoiding needless alarm, which we know to have been the cause of some fatal events both with chloroform and with ether. Such has been my practice since I first obtained the office of full surgeon to a large hospital twenty-one years ago, and I have never had reason to regret it."

Thus he expressed the soundness of his previously expressed views on chloroform but straightway went on to describe a death which occurred in his own private practice while his patient was under chloroform given by Mr. Watson Cheyne. (Cheyne, himself, had "blinkered" views on dangers of chloroform and strenuously opposed Guthrie's suggestions about delayed chloroform poisoning.) The Registrar-General's figures for England and Wales show that in 1882 there were thirty deaths under chloroform, and only one under ether.

Lister then reviewed a number of researches and observations on what did, or did not, constitute a safe concentration of chloroform for the induction of anaesthesia and for its smooth maintenance. At the time it was usual to anaesthetise the patient and to discontinue the administration until signs of consciousness returned whereupon more anaesthetic was given. This was repeated as often as necessary and the whole process meant that surgical conditions were poor and the patient breathed widely varying concentrations of chloroform. Lister also admitted that the use of a folded towel held over the patient's mouth and on to which chloroform is dropped made it impossible for steady concentrations of the agent to be inhaled.

"If for the fitful mode of administration by the folded towel, with atmospheres perpetually oscillating between the needlessly strong and the uselessly weak, we can substitute a method which shall give a uniform and at the same time a mild anaesthetic air, we may anticipate very beneficial results."

He then considered the advantages and disadvantages of the Junker's inhaler and such devices as the Skinner's mask; this was followed by a surprisingly detailed analysis of some rather dubiously based observations and opinions. As a result, Lister reverted to "the corner of a towel, pursed up systematically into a concave mask to cover the mouth and nose by pinching it together at such a distance from the corner that, when the pinched-up part is held over the root of the nose, the corner extends freely to the point of the chin". The mask area, thus produced, varied with the area of the face and, hopefully, with the size of the patient. Chloroform was dropped on to the mask so that its centre was kept moist, but its edges were kept dry, and when induction was accomplished the chloroform drip rate was reduced to half that previously required.

"This method is a little more troublesome than our old plan of holding a folded towel over the face, and replenishing it with chloroform at considerable intervals; but the constant attention which it necessitates is an additional element of safety. During the last five months I have proceeded on these principles, and I have been much pleased with the results."

The method really was not that much different from the folded towel, and the need for the administrator to consider the rate of administration of chloroform by "constant attention" would, according to Lister's earlier writings, have been an unnecessary and dangerous distraction since it conflicted with the over-riding duty to observe the pattern of respiration from breath to breath. Nonetheless, he continued:

"If chloroform given in the simple manner above recommended is really as safe a means of producing prolonged anaesthesia as we possess, a conviction that such is the case will be a great relief to the majority of our practitioners throughout the country; all special apparatus being avoided, and selection of cases needless. For chloroform, if we are once satisfied of its safety, has the grand advantage that it may be used alike for the infant and the aged, and for those affected with pulmonary, cardiac, or renal disease. Wherever an anaesthetic is demanded, chloroform is applicable."

Lister still considered that collapse under chloroform could only be due to idiosyncrasy, or "to want of due watchfulness in the administrator". In such circumstances he believed that Nélaton's head-down position for resuscitation was of value, and that Sylvester's method of artificial respiration was effective. He did not believe that the use of chloroform mixed with alcohol and ether had any advantages over chloroform, and thought that the administration of morphia before chloroform was dangerous. "I understand . . . that a very serious depressing influence upon the nervous system has been sometimes found to result from this combination of the two narcotics". He also mentioned the induction of anaesthesia with nitrous oxide prior to maintenance with ether and thought this to be useful since it spared the patient the unpleasant induction with ether. However, since it involved the inconvenience of bulky apparatus he thought that it would only be of use to dentists, and "to persons who devote themselves specially to the administration of anaesthetics". Such specialists, of course, he thought unnecessary. He also mentioned, briefly, ethidene dichloride and bichloride of methylene but, to him, they had no advantage over his favoured chloroform.

The three articles written by Lister appeared as a chapter in *A System of Surgery* edited by T. Holmes of St. George's Hospital and J. W. Hulke of the Middlesex Hospital in London.[1] The chapter was entitled "Anaesthetics" but this was a misnomer since it did not range over the whole subject in a useful or critical fashion. Instead it consisted, mainly, of anecdotes and platitudes in support of chloroform.

Considering Lister's vast intellectual and practical achievements in other fields his account of anaesthetics displays an attitude which is quite astonishing. It was inept, futile, ill-informed and bigoted. Nonetheless, at the time most practitioners would have paid great attention to the views put forward by one who had, most deservedly, attained eminence because of his brilliant and revolutionary ideas about surgical practice.

With the benefit of hindsight we know that an uncritical eulogy of chloroform was often an epitaph for a patient.

―――――――

A footnote :—

In 1871 Joseph Clover criticised some of Lister's *ex cathedra* statements made about chloroform in an earlier edition of *A System of Surgery* — that is in instalments One and Two to which I have referred above. Clover stated that he had never found it necessary to pull out the tongue, a manoeuvre which, as practised at that date, was a most brutal business using tongue-damaging forceps.[3]

"It is my habit when giving anaesthetics to watch the pulse as well as the breathing, and I am, therefore, better able to speak of the effect of chloroform upon the heart than those who disregard the pulse. It appears that in Mr. Lister's practice the necessity for dragging forward the tongue is of frequent occurrence. Either his method of giving chloroform is not the best that may be devised for preventing the choking, or else the severe process of seizing the tongue with artery-forceps when the choking occurs is not so imperative as he supposes. Probably some of his patients were so affected by the pungency of the vapour that the simple expedient of raising the chin well away from the sternum, which I have never found to fail, might have been sufficient."

For most of his 7,000 chloroform anaesthetics Clover had used his bag apparatus filled with an accurately-prepared mixture of chloroform in air. Joseph Lister replied:[4]

". . . when Mr. Clover attributes his great success to a special apparatus, and when, by proclaiming his own example, he practically counsels medical men in general to disregard the drawing forward of the tongue, he makes, as I believe, a great mistake, and with the best intentions, promulgates most mischievous doctrine. . . . When, therefore, Mr. Clover virtually recommends medical men generally to follow him in abstaining from this practice, he gives about as pernicious a piece of advice as can well be given with reference to the administration of chloroform."

He regarded Clover's apparatus as a "harmless luxury" and pointed out that his own experience was of some 3,500 cases in which the chloroform had been given by young, inexperienced men who did not spend more than three months giving anaesthetics. This was, clearly, a more severe test of the safety of the method than was Clover's own experience in which "the undivided attention of the most experienced special chloroformist in the country was bestowed upon the administration".

"If I devoted my exclusive attention to the administration of the chloroform, I should, for aught I know to the contrary, draw the tongue forward as seldom as he."

So, in 1871, Lister did acknowledge that special experience and expertise could ensure better and safer anaesthesia with chloroform. Why he continued to deny its importance is a mystery.

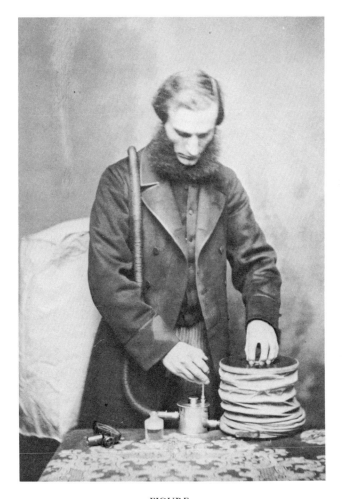

FIGURE 51

Joseph Thomas Clover filling the reservoir bag, slung over his shoulder, with an accurate mixture of $4\frac{1}{2}$ per cent. chloroform in air.

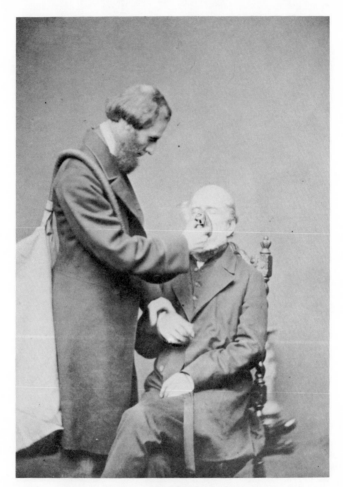

FIGURE 52

Clover, administering chloroform with his apparatus, took great care to feel the pulse during the anaesthetic. Clover was the leading London anaesthetist of his day, being practical, inventive, skilful and scientific. He, not Joseph Lister, should have been asked to write the section on anaesthetics in Holmes and Hulke's *System of Surgery* in 1861. How different it would have been had he done so.

REFERENCES

[1] Holmes, T Hulke, J. W. (1883) *A System of Surgery.* London: Longmans, Green and Co.

[2] Sykes, W. S., (1960) *Essays on the First Hundred Years of Anaesthesia. Volume I,* London, Livingstone.

[3] Clover, J. T. (1871) Chloroform accidents. *British Medical Journal,* **2**, 33–34.

[4] Lister, J. (1871) Chloroform accidents. *British Medical Journal,* **2**, 117–119.

CHAPTER 11

GUTHRIE AND THE CHILDREN:
DELAYED CHLOROFORM POISONING

Leonard George Guthrie was born on the 7th February, 1858, was educated at King's College School and then went on to Magdalen College, Oxford and St. Bartholomew's Hospital, London. He qualified as a doctor in 1888 and, soon afterwards, was appointed House Surgeon to the Paddington Green Children's Hospital. Thereafter, he took a particular interest in the diseases of children, and combined this with a special study of neurological disease. Later, he was appointed to the staff of the Hospital for Epilepsy and Paralysis at Maida Vale in London. He had many interests during his professional career and wrote authoritative, and occasionally witty, papers on children's diseases, nervous disorders and on the history of medicine.

"He had a lofty conception of the position of a physician, and throughout his busy life there was no occasion on which he allowed private advantage to come between him and the high ideals to which he aspired. . . . Those who knew him well were astonished at the multiplicity of his interests, each of which had a share in the development of his mind and character. He was always learning and always developing, and the possibilities of his future seemed even greater than the records of his past, when the end came."[1]

He died on Christmas Eve, 1918 following an accident the previous day. Neither of his two principal, medical obituaries[1,2] mentioned that aspect of his work for which anaesthesia was, and still remains, indebted. For it was Leonard Guthrie who first systematically recorded the series of observations which he had made on a very serious condition which followed chloroform anaesthesia, and which affected children more commonly than adults. He, more than anyone else, established the importance of "delayed chloroform poisoning" and this work, together with that of Goodman Levy a few years later, eventually sealed the fate of chloroform as an anaesthetic.

(It is a strange coincidence that another man with the same surname, but unrelated — Simon Guthrie — had, in New York, been one of the co-discoverers of chloroform in 1831.[3])

There may have been — there almost certainly were — scattered references to the harmful, but delayed effects of chloroform before Leonard Guthrie first drew widespread attention to them in January, 1894.[4,5] However, I have not come across many such reports. One was in 1888,

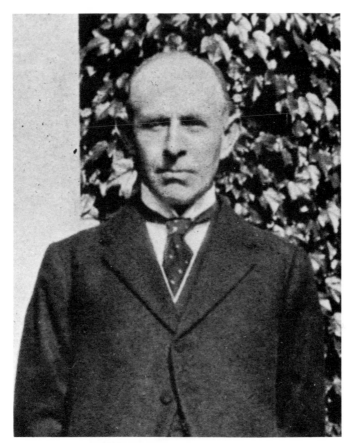

FIGURE 53
Leonard George Guthrie 1858–1918.

when *The Lancet* published an editorial on the dangers of chloroform.[6] The leader deplored the virtual eclipse of the far safer anaesthetic, sulphuric ether, and said:

"Amongst others, the following causes have led to a nearly universal adoption of chloroform, or some chloroform-containing compounds, as the routine anaesthetic in general practice. The mere 'getting a person under' is easy of accomplishment when chloroform is used, and needs little apparatus beyond a drop bottle and a folded towel, and this is a matter of no slight importance to the busy practitioner. And, further, owing to the lamentable absence of instruction in the methods of adminstering anaesthetics, few students gain any experience in the modern modes of procedure, and are quite incompetent to etherise a patient in a satisfactory manner; they find chloroform pretty easy, and so adopt it. But another agency at work has been the strong predilection among Scotch surgeons for chloroform, and the unhesitating manner in which the advantages of that anaesthetic have been paraded, while its dangers have been discounted. These causes have reacted so powerfully to establish chloroform's supposed superiority over ether that it will probably take years before it is at all widely recognised that ether is not only a safer general anaesthetic than chloroform, but is not really difficult to manage if once the method of its administration is mastered. In general, we may affirm that the dangers of chloroform are of such a kind that the utmost human forethought is powerless to avert them, while the disadvantages possessed by ether may usually be wholly obviated by due prevision and careful management of the drug."

Referring to deaths associated with a, generally, uncritical attitude to chloroform's use the leader continued:

"But what is still more unsatisfactory about the results of the crowner's quest in these cases is that we rarely, if ever, find the simple question put, 'Was there any reason why ether could not have been administered instead of chloroform?' . . . In the case of human beings death occurs at three stages: there may be that terrible and sudden dissolution which follows the few initial inbreathings of vapour; while, in the second stage, death is usually said to be due to paralysis of the respiratory centre; and, in the third, it does not take place till some hours after inhalation."

This late death was, it had been suggested, associated with fatty degeneration of the heart, kidneys and liver. The following year, Dr. Robert Ostertag publicised the results of his researches, at the Berlin Pathological Institute, to discover whether or not chloroform could have any "remote effects" when given by inhalation; he concluded that prolonged adminis-trations could be followed by fatty degeneration of organs, which resulted (in susceptible individuals) from the action of chloroform on the blood and upon the tissue cells.[7]

Clearly there was then only limited — albeit potentially powerful — recognition that chloroform may have been a cause of death after its inhalation had ceased. But it was Leonard Guthrie who, in 1894, put the syndrome of delayed chloroform poisoning firmly on the map. His long article, published in two parts,[4,5] covered fifteen columns of solid print and described ten cases (all of them children) in detail; nine of them were fatal.

It is a classic of clear-cut, meticulous observation and careful description, and it brought out into the full light of day a hidden and insidious menace which had almost entirely, and effectively, escaped notice during the forty-seven years or so since chloroform was first introduced as an anaesthetic. We must remember that it was the exception, rather than the rule, for careful records of anaesthesia to be made or kept in those days; the comparatively long incubation period of the condition meant that its connection with the actual anaesthetic would not have been, immediately, obvious. Guthrie, however, who was both physician and pathologist at the Paddington Green Children's Hospital and, having earlier been its chloroformist, was, with his wisdom and perspicacity, well-placed to identify the course of events which sometimes followed chloroform anaesthesia for what they were.

The paper, uncompromisingly entitled "On some fatal after-effects of chloroform in children" began with a description of the usual, benign — but not entirely comfortable — post-anaesthetic course in children, during which vomiting was frequent but rarely prolonged. Guthrie then referred to those rare instances in which the post-chloroform vomiting was prolonged, and recommended the administration of nutrient enemata which, together with a variety of other remedies, were often successful in ending the disorder.

"The symptoms did not recur, and ... no evil consequences ensued, but occasionally screaming and vomiting become symptoms of the gravest import. In this paper ten such cases, nine of which were fatal, are recorded and discussed. The condition in these cases resembles that of acute delirious mania. Shrill, piercing screams are uttered at short intervals. The eyes are dry, the pupils often dilated; the face is sometimes flushed, sometimes pale, and has a look of wild terror and anxiety. There are almost always great restlessness and sleeplessness, the patient tossing and struggling, and requiring constant attention lest the dressings should be torn off or fractured bones displaced. Consciousness is sometimes lost early and in some cases is never regained; but, as a rule, there are intervals in which the child appears to be dull and apathetic, yet answers rationally when addressed and usually denies that it is in pain. ... Vomiting of an extremely violent, copious, and persistent type is an all but invariable symptom. ... In its incessancy and in the volume and character of the vomit it resembles precisely the vomiting which accompanies cerebral disease. . . . The temperature usually undergoes several moderate rises and falls and is commonly above normal at the time of death. . . . Death, as a rule, is owing to gradual exhaustion, the screams become less powerful and are uttered at longer intervals, the vomiting is less violent, unconsciousness leads to coma, respiration and pulse gradually fail, the latter often being imperceptible for a considerable time before the breathing ceases."

Guthrie then presented detailed case reports of ten children who had this severe pattern of illness after chloroform anaesthesia in two of London's children's hospitals — the Paddington Green Children's Hospital and The North Eastern Hospital for Children at the Hackney Road in the East End of London. Nine out of the ten children died, but one survived and made a complete recovery. His first case occurred in November 1887 and the other nine during the next five and a half years. The ten children, whose ages ranged from one to eight and a half years, underwent operations for the drainage of psoas or iliac abscesses, orthopaedic correction of tuberculous or rickety disease and clubbed feet, suprapubic cystostomy for stone and for the radical cure of a hydrocoele. A depressing list, which says much about the general condition of the capital's children at the time. Nonetheless, nearly all the ten children were judged to be in a reasonable general condition on admission to hospital. One, however, was anaemic and had albuminuria. The one child in the series who survived is difficult to discuss; she was eight and a half years old and had a psoas abscess associated with a lumbar spinal curvature. No comment was made about her general condition on admission to hospital, and there is no mention of the anaesthetic agent used or of the duration of the operation. In each of the other case reports chloroform is specifically mentioned as being the anaesthetic agent used, although its duration of administration is not always given. Of the recorded durations, the shortest was 15 minutes, three were of one hour, one of 70 minutes; one operation "was a lengthy one". The deaths occurred, usually, between 10 and 30 hours after the operations, but in one instance it was 53 hours later, and in another the patient lived for six days. Necropsies were performed on eight of the nine patients who died. In three the livers were judged to be normal, but in the other five were described as "pale", "fatty" or "greasy".

Guthrie then proceeded to list the several possible causes of the fatal sequence which he had described, and to discuss their respective pros and cons. His list consisted of "shock with excitement", carbolic acid poisoning, iodoform and mercury poisoning, fat embolism, and the pre-existing pathological conditions of the patients. He felt able, by careful analysis of each patient's clinical condition and progress, to absolve any of these from being the prime causative factor and, having done so, went on:

"The question whether these deaths can be attributed to the remote pathological effects of chloroform must next be considered."

He then reviewed the opinion of many authorities — which had gone unnoticed — to support the contention that chloroform may kill a patient not only instantly, or during its administration, but also hours, days or weeks after its administration, and discussed the applicability of these various opinions to the events which befell his nine young patients, with particular emphasis on the impairment of liver function which seemed to him to be the most important factor.

"Will the condition of the liver account for the symptoms in these cases of death following operations? Seeing that the symptoms of fatty liver are practically unknown — and under other circumstances I am not aware that any deaths have ever been attributed to this condition alone — the question is a difficult one to decide. The symptoms in these cases are of pronounced cerebral type, and in this respect they resemble those of acute yellow atrophy of the liver or phosphorus poisoning. . . . Theoretical though the explanation may be, I am unable to account otherwise for these fatalities after operation than by supposing: 1) that these deaths . . . were due to auto-intoxication: 2) that a fatty condition of the liver and therefore functional disturbance of the organ existed before the operations; and 3) that chloroform and operation shock combined aggravated the condition already present and thus loaded the system with toxic alkaloids which the kidneys . . . were unable to eliminate. The practical results of such views are: 1) that in no case should chloroform be given to patients suffering from fatty liver; 2) that as it is impossible from physical signs and symptoms to do more than surmise the existence of fatty liver we must rely on signs of functional inactivity of the liver, as indicated by the excess of alkaloidal substances present in the urine; and 3) that the precise nature of such alkaloidal substances and the best methods of detecting them must be left for further investigation."

For good measure, he added "The mortality in these cases shows the futility of the treatment adopted . . ."

A week later a letter from W. Watson Cheyne, who had been the surgeon in charge of five of the cases described by Guthrie, was published.[8] He disagreed entirely with Guthrie's interpretation of the events. One of his cases, he suggested, was clearly a case of fat embolism following an osteotomy, and another had been caused by carbolic acid poisoning since the patient had passed olive-green urine, which was typical of that condition. However, he brought forward no conclusive evidence to prove that these were the principal causes of death in these two instances. The death of another of the cases he ascribed firmly to fat embolism; there were no real signs of this condition, but the patient did have carboluria which, for some reason, Watson Cheyne did not think was important this time. He gave no reasons for his inconsistency. In yet another case, in which carbolic acid had not been used at all, death was ascribed to fat embolism, but this must have been somewhat far-fetched, since the patient had had an iliac abscess drained. He then went on to say that he no longer used carbolic acid so freely and, since making this change, no more deaths had occurred. (I cannot really believe that Watson Cheyne thought that the lesser use of carbolic acid would prevent both carboluria and fat embolism, but that is one interpretation of what he had said.) He concluded his letter:

"I do not, of course, deny the existence of serious and fatal effects after anaesthetics; indeed I believe they are not uncommon, especially after ether. In fact I think that, if the after-effects of ether are taken into sufficient consideration there will not be much to choose between it and chloroform in point of view of danger. I would even go so far as to say that if the use of chloroform were entirely prohibited, as was at one time strongly hinted at in some of the journals, and if ether were used in all instead of only in suitable cases, as at present, its death-roll (including its after-effects) would be as great as, and probably greater than, that of chloroform."

It would have been well if Watson Cheyne had taken the advice which John Hunter had given to Jenner. "Don't think. Try the experiment."

A week later, *The Lancet's* leader pointed out the importance of Guthrie's observations and, fairly, stated that his views could hardly be accepted as conclusive.[9] Clearly, contrary views had been expressed by Watson Cheyne, and the Hyderabad Chloroform Commission's findings did not lend credence to Guthrie's opinions.

"But, whether Dr. Guthrie be right or wrong in the extent to which he has assigned the influence of chloroform in those cases, he deserves thanks for bringing this important subject under notice. It is hardly possible for the matter to end here. It is not a mere record of some singular phenomena in the history of surgical operations. It is a grave indictment against the use of a most valuable adjuvant to the armamentarium of the surgeon. . . . Once more we urge the need for research and inquiry, and invite the attention of our leading medical societies to a subject fraught with grave and important issues."

Guthrie did not write further about the condition until some nine years later.[10] He reported four more cases to *The Lancet* and said that in none of these could fat embolism or carbolic acid poisoning be considered as causes of the fatalities. Three of the patients had been children and one was an adult aged 41 years. As before he discussed the case reports in meticulous detail and considered, most carefully, the differential diagnoses. Again, he came, in all important respects, to the same conclusions at which he had arrived in his earlier papers. Some comment on the rarity of the condition may be made since Guthrie, favourably situated as he was in a children's hospital, had taken seven years to collect his first series of ten cases, and a further nine years to collect another four. I have no doubt that other, similar cases must have occurred but, for some reason, they were not recognised for what they were; perhaps, some of those which were correctly diagnosed were kept from Guthrie. After all, chloroform was a very popular and highly thought of anaesthetic agent for most of the time over which his observations ranged.

Shortly after Guthrie's second set of observations W. P. Montgomery wrote that:

"The paper opens up a most important question, for I fancy that most surgeons in children's practice have had the misfortune to lose cases within 48 hours of a comparatively simple operation and after the succession of symptoms described."[11]

Dr. Montgomery then described the case of a three-year-old boy who had died after chloroform anaesthesia for a hernia operation performed at the Manchester Children's Hospital. The clinical course was like those described by Guthrie, and carbolic acid had not been used as an antiseptic. Watson Cheyne would have been hard put to attribute this disaster to fat embolism or carbolic acid poisoning.

In 1904, Mr. Harold Stiles and Dr. Stuart McDonald, both of Edinburgh, presented a paper to a special meeting of the Society for the Study of Disease in Children on what had, by then, become known as "Delayed Chloroform Poisoning".[12] They pointed out that the condition had been recognised in adults, in Germany, for some time but acknowledged that it was Guthrie, with his painstaking and persistent work, who had highlighted the disorder in the United Kingdom. They then described two more fatal cases in children, and deduced that, in these, the chloroform anaesthesia had been the crucial factor, although they felt that it was, then, impossible to prove or disprove Guthrie's suggestion. Watson Cheyne, who was chairman of the meeting, had obviously begun to modify his views and said that "he was still not quite convinced that chloroform was the only causative factor". Leonard Guthrie had no doubts and still avowed that the chloroform was the most important feature, and thought that its role was that of a "last straw" in the presence of pre-existing liver disease which, he said, was difficult to diagnose.

Dr. J. F. W. Silk, of King's College Hospital, London waggishly declared himself now to be

"very astonished to find that it had been discovered in Edinburgh of all places that quite possibly chloroform might produce some ill-effects."

A year later, E. W. Scott Carmichael, an Edinburgh surgeon, with one of his pathologist colleagues, Dr. James Beattie, described another case of delayed chloroform poisoning in a three-year-old child who had died 42 hours after operation and at post mortem was found to have a fatty, yellow liver.[13] They also summed up most of the doubts which, then, existed about the exact cause of the condition.

"Guthrie has maintained that in these cases the chloroform has acted merely as a helper on of a pre-existing process. The very small number of deaths as compared with the number of chloroform anaesthesias gives some support to this view. Still, though we cannot disprove his contention we agree with those who maintain that the condition is a primary one and wholly due to the chloroform. It has been shown conclusively by experiments on animals that this extreme fatty degeneration can be produced in healthy organs after subcutaneous injection of chloroform."

At the end of 1905, the "Annus Medicus", which was *The Lancet's* yearly review of current practice, mentioned an American report by Dr. James A. Kelly of Boston, Massachusetts.[14] In 400 cases operated upon under chloroform 46 had shown symptoms of "acid intoxication", and, of these, six had died. The syndrome, at the time, was widely believed to be due to an acidic chemical toxaemia with acetone and diacetic acid. Dr. Kelly described the symptoms very much as Guthrie had observed; in those cases which went to post mortem the livers had resembled those seen in acute yellow atrophy. The following year, three more fatal cases of delayed chloroform poisoning were reported by Mr. E. D. Telford and Dr. J. L. Falconer of the Manchester Hospital for Sick Children.[15] They pointed out that the condition had first been described in 1850 and, by 1906, some 70 cases had been reported. Many of the cases had occurred in children with rickets and this, they thought, might have been an important predisposing cause. They added:

"It may, of course, be objected that rickets supplies a very large proportion of the operative work of any children's hospital. . . ."

which, again, is a very revealing and depressing comment upon the state of children's health at the beginning of the twentieth century.

This account stimulated Leonard Guthrie to write again to *The Lancet.*[16] This time he pointed out, *inter alia*, that delayed anaesthetic poisoning had occurred not only after chloroform but also, to a lesser extent, with ether. This, Guthrie reasoned,

". . . lends support to the view that the pre-disposing cause of delayed poisoning by chloroform and other anaesthetics is a pre-existing and morbidly fatty condition of the liver. For although it is without dispute that prolonged inhalation of chloroform will induce extreme fatty changes, ether is only capable of inducing them to an infinitesimal extent. Therefore, if a markedly fatty liver is found in fatal ether cases it follows that it must have been fatty before the inhalation. . . .

"Granting the existence of a liver overcharged with fat, it is not difficult to imagine that the effect of a general anaesthetic, especially chloroform, may be as the 'last straw' . . ."

He then summarised his own views on safe practice as far as chloroform was concerned.

"The practical outcome of the opinions which I have imperfectly expressed are: 1. Operations should be delayed when possible if a fatty liver be suspected. It may be suspected in subjects of rickets and infantile paralysis who have been overfed with fattening food and under-exercised; in cases of sepsis and diabetes, and when a history of cyclical vomiting is obtained. 2. When a child has recently vomited apparently without cause, an intended operation should be postponed. This precaution has been neglected in many fatal cases recorded. 3. When fatty liver is suspected the patient should be kept for some days on a diet restricted in fats and starch. 4. Bicarbonate of soda should be given meanwhile in order to neutralise fatty acids which may be present. 5. Starvation and fright will both give rise to acute acetonuria. The effects of fright may to some extent be combated by avoiding starvation. Nutrient enemata should be given two hours before and immediately after an operation. 6. Although any general anaesthetic may be dangerous in the presence of a fatty liver, chloroform is most dangerous of all on account of its specific action on the liver and kidneys."

H. H. B. Cunningham then reported, from Belfast, a case diagnosed as "acid intoxication" after ethyl chloride.[17] A girl of six was given the anaesthetic for one minute for the removal of her adenoids. She made an apparently normal recovery, but began to vomit the next day. She had headache, diacetic acid in the urine and relapsed into a "typhoid state". She was treated with bicarbonate of soda and recovered. It is more than somewhat doubtful whether this was a genuine case.

But eight more, genuine, cases occurred during 1908. No less than four of these appeared in one number of *The Lancet*. Henry Thorp, of Stafford, described the first.[18] A child, nearly four years old, was circumcised; the operation lasted 7 minutes and two drachms of chloroform were used. He died in just over 36 hours, some 23 hours after the first symptoms appeared.

Mr. E. D. Telford wrote again to *The Lancet* and reported three more cases, all in rickety children.[19] Two of these died; the third "recovered from an apparently hopeless position". T. M. Bride reported two more cases from the Manchester Children's Hospital; both children were rickety and one of them died.[20] Hugh C. Wilson, then House Surgeon at the Paddington Green Children's Hospital reported another fatal case,[21] as did Dr. Mary Taylor,[22] who wrote from Rome about a case she had looked after as house physician at the Belgrave Hospital for Children, in London.

Dr. A. P. Beddard, a physician at Guy's and the West London Hospitals, made some suggestions for the treatment of the condition in 1908.[23] He reasoned:

"It would seem worth while to try feeding such patients with dextrose either by the mouth, or failing this by enemata or continuous rectal infusion of a 10 to 20 per cent solution or even by infusing intravenously a 6 per cent solution."

and particularly advised this regime before chloroform anaesthesia in rickety or other, ill-nourished children. Another London physician also came to this conclusion.[24] Dr. William Hunter argued his case carefully, and came to the conclusion that

"The vomiting which occurs after administration of anaesthetics is not of nervous origin; but it is, I consider, essentially toxaemic, due to the profound depression of liver function with consequent diminution in its antitoxic function during the period of administration. This depression will be greater if a liver already weakened by disease or by poor nutrition be further unduly weakened by food having been witheld for many hours before the administration. This enforced abstention from food before administration of an anaesthetic may thus in individual cases be carried too far, and it is, in my opinion, largely responsible for the fatal effects of delayed chloroform poisoning in exceptional cases. Such effects could in all probability be prevented if, instead of witholding food, particular care was taken that the patient had always a very nutritious and easily digestible meal, well-sweetened, two or three hours before operation."

In 1909, T. C. Somerville had three cases in Huddersfield. Two happened in adults, and all three patients died.[25] In London, W. H. Payne was more fortunate. The three cases which he had diagnosed as delayed chloroform poisoning all recovered. He attributed the cause of the initial damage to "acetone chloroform" which was a more cheaply made preparation than that usually used. He, thereafter, used only the most pure chemical and claimed to have eliminated the problem by so doing.[26] Dr. A. A. Weir wrote from Australia of a case which recovered, but it seems doubtful if delayed chloroform poisoning was the correct diagnosis, since vomiting was virtually absent.[27] An annotation in *The Lancet* recorded another fatal case, first reported by Drs. Whipple and Sperry at the Johns Hopkins Hospital in Baltimore, and went on to suggest that chloroform could be most safely used if it was given in accurately metered and minimal doses to patients who were kept in good general condition throughout the period of anaesthesia.[28]

Yet again, Mr. E. D. Telford wrote from Manchester to make several apt and accurate observations.[29] He first described the case of one of his adult patients, aged 47 who had a gastro-enterostomy for pyloric obstruction under chloroform anaesthesia. At the time of the operation the liver looked and felt absolutely normal. She developed all the features of delayed chloroform poisoning after operation and, at post mortem, her liver was found to be slightly enlarged, bright yellow and fatty. This argued against Guthrie's theory that prior liver disease or damage was important. Telford then wrote:

"Cases such as the above form a very strong indictment against the indiscriminate use of chloroform. Since my last report of cases of 'delayed chloroform poisoning' I have used ether in almost every case . . . given by the 'open' method from an Allis inhaler after a preliminary induction of anaesthesia by ethyl chloride. . . . No untoward after-effect has ever been noted. Lastly, it will be found that with increasing experience the supposed limitations of ether as an anaesthetic will recede almost to vanishing point."

Other reports and observations were published; some were informative, others were not.[30,31,32,33,34,35] There was not, really, very much that anyone could add to Mr. Telford's comments. The only way to avoid delayed chloroform poisoning with absolute certainty was to avoid chloroform absolutely. Deaths from the condition were rare and not so spectacular or dramatic as those of sudden heart failure. But the patients were just as dead.

REFERENCES

[1] Obituary (1919) *British Medical Journal,* **1**, 28–29.
[2] Obituary (1919) *Lancet,* **1**, 44.
[3] Snow, J. (1858) *On Chloroform and other Anaesthetics.* London: Churchill.
[4] Guthrie, L. G. (1894) On some fatal after-effects of chloroform on children. *Lancet,* **1**, 193–197.
[5] Guthrie, L. G. (1894) On some fatal after-effects of chloroform on children. *Lancet,* **1**, 257–261.
[6] Editorial (1888) *Lancet,* **2**, 523–524.
[7] Anonymous. (1889) The pathological effects of chloroform inhalation. *Lancet,* **2**, 1072.
[8] Cheyne, W. W. (1894) The after-effects of chloroform. *Lancet,* **1**, 370.
[9] Editorial (1894) *Lancet,* **1**, 419–420.

[10] Guthrie, L. G. (1903) On the fatal effects of chloroform on children suffering from a peculiar condition of fatty liver. *Lancet*, **2**, 10–17.

[11] Montgomery, W. P. (1903) The fatal effects of chloroform on children suffering from a peculiar condition of fatty liver. *Lancet* **3**, 267.

[12] Anonymous (1904) Delayed chloroform poisoning. *Lancet*, **1**, 1657–1659.

[13] Scott Carmichael, E. W., Beattie, J. M. (1905) Delayed chloroform poisoning. *Lancet*, **2**, 437–440.

[14] Anonymous (1905) The Annus Medicus. *Lancet*, **2**, 1900–1946.

[15] Telford, E. D., Falconer, J. L. (1906) Delayed chloroform poisoning. *Lancet*, **2**, 1341–1343.

[16] Guthrie, L. G. (1906) Delayed chloroform poisoning. *Lancet*, **2**, 1542–1543.

[17] Cunningham, H. H. B. (1908) Acid intoxication following ethyl-chloride anaesthesia. *Lancet*, **1**, 284–285.

[18] Thorp, H. (1908) A case of acid intoxication following the administration of chloroform. *Lancet*, **1**, 623.

[19] Telford, E. D. (1908) Three cases of delayed chloroform poisoning. *Lancet*, **1**, 623–624.

[20] Bride, T. M. (1908) A report on two cases of delayed chloroform toxaemia. *Lancet*, 2, 625–626.

[21] Wilson, H. C. (1908) A fatal case of delayed chloroform poisoning. *Lancet*, **1**, 626–627.

[22] Taylor, M. F. (1908) Fatal toxaemia after administration of chloroform. *Lancet*, **2**, 799–800.

[23] Beddard, A. P. (1908) A suggestion for treatment in delayed chloroform poisoning. *Lancet*, **1**, 782–783.

[24] Hunter, W. (1908) Delayed chloroform poisoning: its nature and prevention. *Lancet*, **1**, 993–995.

[25] Somerville, T. C. (1909) Three cases of delayed chloroform poisoning. *Lancet*, **2**, 81–82.

[26] Payne, W. H. (1909) Delayed chloroform poisoning. *Lancet*, **2**, 187.

[27] Weir, A. A. (1909) A case of "delayed chloroform poisoning" treated with dextrose; recovery. *Lancet*, **2**, 710.

[28] Anonymous (1909) Delayed poisoning after chloroform inhalation. *Lancet*, **2**, 1608.

[29] Telford, E. D. (1910) Some notes on "delayed chloroform poisoning". *Lancet*, **2**, 1269–1270.

[30] Clark, G. H. (1911) The influence of chloroform when repeatedly administered in small doses. *Lancet*, **1**, 158–161.

[31] Anonymous (1912) Post-anaesthetic poisoning. *Lancet*, **1**, 1130–1131.

[32] Clark, G. H. (1912) The distribution of chloroform in the blood. *Lancet*, **2**, 235–236.

[33] Anonymous (1912) *Lancet*, **2**, 524–525.

[34] Fairlie, H. P. (1914) A case of delayed chloroform poisoning. *Lancet*, **2**, 1411–1412.

[35] Todd, T. F. (1934) Delayed chloroform poisoning *Lancet*, **2**, 597–598.

CHAPTER 12

A VERY BUSY THIRTY-THREE DAYS

Sir William Mitchell Banks, surgeon to the Liverpool Royal Infirmary, wrote a long, ten-column article entitled "Impressions about chloroform and ether" in 1901.[1] He said that he had given all of Professor Syme's hospital anaesthetics in Edinburgh for six months; this would have given a small experience of about 150 cases,[2] and a very strong and lasting conviction that he knew all about anaesthesia. He then gave chloroform in Liverpool to nearly all of Mr. Edward Bickersteth's private patients for six years, and saw all the operations performed at the Royal Infirmary. Mitchell Banks then made a careful calculation of the extent of his experience at the time he wrote the article. He had been in Liverpool for over 34 years, and reckoned he had had 42 working weeks in each year, with an average of six cases a week. This made the total, according to him, of about 8,500 cases. I checked his arithmetic — for reasons which will appear shortly — and found that, in this instance, it was approximately correct. The exact figure was 8,568. He referred to his cases in Liverpool only but, in order to give him every possible advantage let us add on Syme's 150 cases to make a total of 8,718.

He then ranged over various subjects, some of which were debatable but reasonable enough.

"What special and particular good came out of the Hyderabad Commission I never could see. There is no possible comparison between a healthy dog or cat or any other animal and a diseased human being. They are not in the least under the same conditions, and experiments upon them are therefore useless. . . . I often speak . . . of the White Man and the Blue Man. The White Man is being poisoned by chloroform and is always in a dangerous way. His heart is working very feebly and at any minute may give out. The Blue Man, it is true, ought not to have been allowed to become blue, but still he is not in such straits as the other. If he can get a little air into his lungs to oxygenate his blood it will still be very hard to kill him."

Sir William then went on to say that he had had two deaths from chloroform, and advised that chloroformists should use only simple apparatus.

"As for those great apparatuses which people wear on their backs (like Parisian lemonade-sellers) or the apparatuses with stopcocks which profess to give regulated quantities of anaesthetics, my notion is that as anaesthetics have to be given in country cottages and in the houses of the poor dwellers in cities as well as in those of the rich, such apparatuses should not be used. The student should be taught to use the simple tools with which he is likely to go into practice."

Surprisingly, as a disciple of Syme, he always made a point of examining the heart before anaesthesia. But, as befitted his origins, he was in no doubt as to who bore the responsibility for the anaesthetic.

"With a few exceptions I cannot say that I have ever felt very anxious about the performance of any surgical operation, because I have never been ashamed to beat a retreat in time if things were going against me. But the anaesthetic always has been and always will be to me a serious source of dread. I have therefore always maintained a careful watch on the progress of the anaesthetisation. . . . I therefore hold that, in the matter of the anaesthetic, the surgeon should be master over the management of that, as over every other detail of the operation."

Most anaesthetists would pity and disagree with Sir William here, knowing the utter futility and impossibility of trying to perform major surgery efficiently at the same time as attempting to supervise the conduct of the anaesthesia. Another sentence of Sir William's would appear to give substantial backing to this opinion, although he would not have admitted it. "In both the chloroform fatalities which I have seen the patient was stone dead by the time my attention was drawn to them". So much for the value of the careful watch, and the mastery of the surgeon over the details. But the best is yet to come. Thirty-three days later Sir William Mitchell Banks spoke at a meeting at the Liverpool Medical Institution. In the course of his address he said

". . . he felt certain that but for his own supervision he would not have seen two deaths out of some 11,000 or 12,000 cases, but more likely 20."[3]

He really and truly believed that his own supervision was effective, in spite of the fact that, on two occasions, it had to be pointed out to him that his patient was dead!

Now, thirty-three days before this address, Mitchell Banks' total anaesthetic experience, according to his own figures, amounted to 8,500 cases; according to my slightly more generous estimate it came to 8,718. So, if his figures are to be believed, during those thirty-three days he must have given at least 2,282, and possibly 3,282, additional anaesthetics in order to bring his total up to the figure which he had quoted to the Liverpool Medical Institution. This means that he must have administered between 69 and 99 anaesthetics on each and every day in the interval, depending on whether we accept his figure of 11,000 anaesthetics given, or prefer his estimate of 12,000.

He must, indeed, have been very busy.

REFERENCES

[1] Banks, W. M. (1901) Impressions about chloroform and ether. *Lancet*, **2**, 1323–1328.

[2] Sykes, W. S. (1960) *Essays on the First Hundred Years of Anaesthesia. Volume I.* Edinburgh: Livingstone.

[3] Anonymous (1902) Liverpool Medical Institution. *Lancet*, **1**, 25–26.

CHAPTER 13

BICHLORIDE OF METHYLENE

Bichloride of methylene (also variously referred to as chloromethyl, methylene chloride, dichloromethane, chlorinated chloride of methyl, methylenic chloride and, often, simply as "methylene") was first used for anaesthesia on the 15th October, 1867 by Benjamin Ward Richardson. The operation, ovariotomy, was performed by Spencer Wells who, over the next four years, operated on patients under methylene 250 times. In 1871 he wrote:

"I have never been at all uneasy in any one of these cases ... whereas with chloroform I never felt quite at ease."[1]

Benjamin Ward Richardson's first suggestion that methylene bichloride could be used for anaesthesia was recorded in the *British Medical Journal*[2] just four days after Spencer Wells' original operation at which Richardson himself had administered his new general anaesthetic. This was in an account of one of his private lectures entitled "Bichloride of Methylene as a General Anaesthetic" which he had delivered on the 8th October, 1867, that is, seven days before he first used the agent clinically; he had, however, inhaled it himself to the point of "perfect insensibility".[1] In his lecture Richardson had reviewed the chemistry of the series chloride of methyl (CH_3Cl), bichloride of methylene (CH_2Cl_2), chloroform ($CHCl_3$) and carbon tetrachloride (CCl_4) which, he said, all possessed anaesthetic properties. He stated that his new agent seemed to be safer than chloroform and proceeded to render three pigeons insensible within glass jars, into which he introduced chloroform, carbon tetrachloride and methylene. He deduced that, when compared to chloroform, his bichloride gave a slower induction and a more rapid, though delayed, awakening.

The following week *The Lancet* published an editorial on the subject.[3]

"Nobody will be surprised to hear of the discovery of a new anaesthetic or that the discoverer is Dr. Richardson. ... Every man has his weak point, and we would just hint to Dr. Richardson, out of regard for his genius, that he is somewhat apt not thoroughly to complete one discovery, and making sure of its being a real one, before hastening in search of another. ...

"We are anxious to get the greatest amount of good and the least amount of disappointment out of it. So while we should like to chain Dr. Richardson down to the completion of one or two practical discoveries, we must take his contributions to science as he pleases to give us them. . . .

"In its action the bichloride of methylene is more gentle, but as effective as chloroform; it produces less struggling and less vascular excitement. Its narcotic effects are equally prolonged. It acts very uniformly on the nervous centres. It produces sometimes vomiting. When it is carried so far as to kill, it destroys by equally paralysing the heart and the respiration. It interferes less than other anaesthetics with the muscular irritability.

"Dr. Richardson expects that it will prove less fatal than chloroform, which causes death, he estimates, once in fifteen hundred cases. He is very right, however, in speaking diffidently on this point, for there are no facts to justify confidence."

Monsieur Tourdes and Monsieur Hepp experimented with bichloride of methylene in Strasbourg and their findings were reviewed in the *British Medical Journal*.[4] They noted that it produced rapid and complete anaesthesia which lasted for several minutes, and that it could be repeated at intervals of 3 to 4 minutes for prolonged procedures. They did not, however, consider that it had any advantage over chloroform, except for cases in which it was felt that a slighter degree of anaesthesia was necessary.

Richard Rendle, of Guy's Hospital, London reported his use of methylene in 1869.[5] He had anaesthetised 40 cases using a Junker's apparatus and had found that in some patients the induction of anaesthesia was unduly prolonged; three patients took 20 minutes to induce. He then reported on a further 123 cases in which he had used his own inhaler and this had greatly reduced the length of induction. (In the same article he also described the use of nitrous oxide given from Barth's iron bottles with Coleman's slaked lime absorber. This gave great economy of gas. With great clinical acumen he kept the expiratory valve on his inhaler open for the first three breaths so as to get rid of much of the nitrogen in the lungs.)

The first death during methylene anaesthesia occurred at the Charing Cross Hospital, London in October, 1869.[6] The anaesthetic was given by Mr. Peter Marshall for a resection of the jaw performed by Mr. Canton. Further details were given a fortnight later.[7] The patient had been a man aged 30 on whom Mr. Canton had refused to operate until the matter was pressed. One drachm (3·6 mls.) of methylene was given in the first three minutes and this was followed by another half drachm (1·8 mls.). The patient, who was in a very feeble condition, then suddenly died. Peter Marshall, who had considerable experience of the use of methylene, gave an account of the case himself.[8] A malignancy involved the left antrum of Highmore and had spread locally; an operation was not considered to be practicable, but the patient and his friends had urged the surgeon to

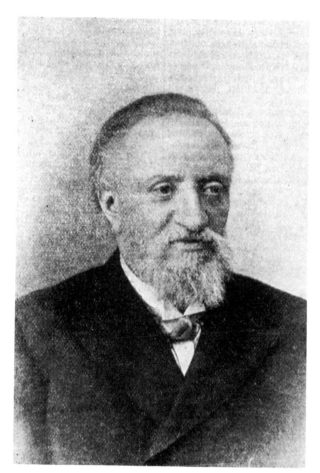

FIGURE 54
Sir Benjamin Ward Richardson, M.D., LL.D., F.R.C.P., F.R.S. 1828–1896.

intervene. The patient had been a very bad risk having been enfeebled by previous haemorrhage, the growth itself and mental depression. He had been anaesthetised sitting in a chair and his respiratory efforts had been hampered by "the necessary bandage round the abdomen to prevent struggling during the operation". Death occurred before the surgery had started.

There was a further annotation of this case in *The Lancet* which had sought the views of Dr. Richardson himself.[9] He said that bichloride of methylene had been given in some six or seven thousand cases with only this one fatal ending.

Richardson wrote another article about methylene in 1869.[10]

"I have written these lines about the bichloride without any desire to praise it because it is an introduction of my own."

This was, without doubt, true: he added a postscript to his article and carefully recorded the death of Peter Marshall's patient. He stressed the patient's grave condition before operation and pointed out that the patient, knowingly, had accepted responsibility for the operation. Anaesthesia was, in fact, a euthanasia.

A second death during methylene chloride anaesthesia occurred in 1871, again at the Charing Cross Hospital.[11] The anaesthetic was given to the patient, a highly nervous, 41-year-old labourer, for the amputation of a finger.

"... the operation not lasting more than one minute. It was then found that the deceased's head had fallen upon one side, his eyes were upturned, and breathing and pulsation had ceased.... There was no doubt that the death of the deceased had been produced by the methylene he had inhaled. The cases of death while under the influence of methylene were extremely rare."

Even so, in 1872 another death occurred, this time at the Middlesex Hospital in London.[12] A 48-year-old man had been admitted for incision of a deep abscess in his buttock.

"Methylene was used on this occasion; about two drachms [7·2 mls.] had been inhaled and he was insensible; when, as the operation was about to be commenced, and a minute after the inhalation had been stopped, it was noticed that his breathing had ceased and he became very livid."

Two more methylene deaths occurred in 1884, one during dental extraction,[13] and one during nerve suture.[14] In the latter case it was said that too much methylene could not be applied at once because it would only evaporate at a certain rate.

These five were the only separately recorded fatalities associated with methylene bichloride that I could find.

In 1878 Spencer Wells spoke enthusiastically on the bichloride of methylene during a lecture delivered at the Royal College of Surgeons of England.

"I have no doubt whatever, myself, from long trial of it, that the bichloride of methylene, as it is called, is a far safer anaesthetic than chloroform. Since I have used it, I believe in more than six hundred cases of ovariotomy and more than three hundred operations of other kinds, I have never once been in the smallest anxiety about a patient. . . . Provided it is carefully given in a proper apparatus, I have never seen the smallest cause for anxiety. This apparatus was contrived by Dr. Junker a good many years ago."[15]

He thought that Junker's apparatus would, at the most, produce a 4 per cent. mixture of the methylene bichloride in air and that it was more usually a 2 per cent. mixture; 4 per cent. in air, he said, was positively safe. He also added that pure methylene bichloride was unstable and began to decompose in half an hour or so. Alcohol was added to confer stability on the mixture but, even so some (not Spencer Wells) considered the liquid used for anaesthesia to be merely a mixture of chloroform and spirit.

F. E. Junker, in 1883, wrote of a death associated with methylene administered with his apparatus to a patient in Prague:

". . . which being the tenth fatal case from this anaesthetic, must considerably shake the confidence of the profession in its perfect safety."[16]

The fluid used for the anaesthesia was examined in Prague and the chemical analyst reported:

"The fluid, which I received in the original bottle, with the label — 'Bichloride of methylene, CH_2Cl_2, manufactured by J. Robbins and Co., Manufacturing and Pharmaceutical Chemists, 147, Oxford Street, London' — was found, on examination, to be a mixture of chloroform and alcohol. . . . the fluid contained either no chloride of methylene at all, or merely traces of it."

The manufacturers, Robbins and Company, then wrote to the *British Medical Journal* to defend their product.[17] They reminded their readers of Junker's own earlier and published enthusiasm for the agent,[18] and it is certainly true that, when Junker described his ingenious apparatus in 1867, he recommended it for use with both chloroform and chloromethyl.[19] Robbins and Co. refuted his suggestion, or rather that of the chemist in Prague, that their bichloride of methylene could possibly be a mixture of chloroform and alcohol. No mixture of these, they said, would make a fluid

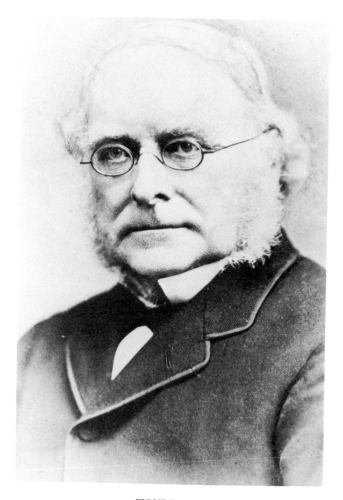

FIGURE 55
Sir Thomas Spencer Wells. He was Richardson's surgical colleague, and thought very highly of "methylene".

like methylene. This substance was made by the action of metallic zinc on a mixture of chloroform and ethyl or methyl alcohol. On heating, chloride of zinc was formed from the chloroform and oxide of zinc from the alcohol; this proved that a chemical change was taking place. The process, it is recorded, was difficult and slow because the zinc became protected from further action by the formation of oxychloride. Dr. Richardson, it was noted, had taken ten days to make just 15 ozs. (426 mls.) in 1867.

All this inspired Dr. Robert Kirk, of Glasgow, to write that the brand of methylene which he usually had used was "Morson's" and that this was excellent. However, he had used some manufactured by Robbin's and this, by and large, he equated with chloroform. He had also arranged for a chemical analysis of the two manufacturers' products; both contained 80 per cent. chloroform. The remainder in Robbin's brand appeared to be methylene chloride and in Morson's was a different substance which he could not identify.[20]

In 1883, the Academy of Medicine of Paris held two meetings in an attempt to shed some light on the dubious chemical composition of the bichloride of methylene which was used for anaesthesia, and on its clinical usefulness. Junker summarised the proceedings of these two meetings in the *British Medical Journal*.[21] The two principals involved were Monsieur Regnauld, Professor of Chemistry in the Faculty of Medicine and Monsieur Léon Le Fort, surgeon to the Hôtel Dieu in Paris.

Monsieur Léon Le Fort had read of Spencer Wells' enthusiasm for chloride of methylene and determined to try it in his own practice for abdominal surgery. Before doing so he asked, wisely, Professeur Regnauld to subject the preparation sold under the name of chloride of methylene by various manufacturing chemists to a careful chemical analysis. Regnauld, who had made a special study of the chemistry of substances used for anaesthesia, failed to discover any trace of "chlorinated chloride of methylene" in any of the samples he had analysed. They consisted, without exception, merely of chloroform together with a small quantity of alcohol (ordinarily used, apparently, in its preservation).

So impressed was Monsieur Le Fort by Spencer Wells' insistence that the new anaesthetic produced far less vomiting than did chloroform after abdominal and gynaecological surgery that he took the matter further.

"I then wrote to Sir Spencer Wells who furnished me with the name and address of his purveyor, from whom I obtained a preparation ... M. Regnauld, after examination, declared that it was not common chloroform, but neither chloride of methyl, the boiling points being different."

Monsieur Le Fort was not much convinced by the results of the chemical analysis which he had commissioned.

"I shall continue with the chloride of methylene . . . it has given me far superior results than the best of our chloroforms."

Regnauld did not, however, wonder at the good effects of this English preparation,

". . . a compound of four parts of chloroform and one of methylic alcohol . . . to which the term bichloride of methylene and the formula CH_2Cl_2 was misapplied."

Methylic alcohol, Regnauld pointed out, had been discovered by the eminent chemist Monsieur Dumas, and it possessed narcotic properties. Monsieur Dumas was present at these meetings of the Academy of Medicine of Paris.

Junker then reported that he had tried, in 20 patients, the mixture of which Regnauld had said that the English methylene bichloride was composed. He found it a most satisfactory anaesthetic.

Spencer Wells returned to the defence of bichloride of methylene in 1890 during the course of another lecture delivered to the Royal College of Surgeons of England. He had, he said, more than 20 years experience of its use as an anaesthetic for a large number of operations, some of which were "exceptionally long".[22] As he had said before, he had the gravest doubts about the safety of chloroform but few, if any, concerning the bichloride of methylene.

In 1896, Sir Benjamin Ward Richardson attempted to sum up the controversy which task, for someone in his particular position, was somewhat difficult.[23] He pointed out that in the early days of anaesthesia deaths had been rarely due to the agents themselves and, had it been otherwise, anaesthesia itself would have probably died out. By 1866 Richardson's own enquiries revealed that 1 in every 2,500 anaesthetics ended in a fatality. Later, in 1870 it had been observed that 1 in 7,000 anaesthetics, using methylene, caused death. For chloroform the figure was 1 in 2,723, for ether 1 in 23,204, and for nitrous oxide it was 1 in 75,000. He concluded that the presence of chlorine atoms in the substance added to its risk as an anaesthetic, and that the greater the number of chlorine atoms in the molecules the greater was the danger to the patient. (This consideration must have occurred to him some time after his first suggestion that bichloride of methylene would be a useful alternative to chloroform; he did not mention it in his original paper in 1867.) His next point was revealing.

"I have always administered methylene, instead of chloroform with success. I treat with the silence it deserves the continental rumour that the great French chemist ... made a specimen of the bichloride from which, in my opinion, the chlorine could not have been properly removed, and which was, therefore, fatal. I treat also with the same silence the widespread absurdity that bichloride of methylene is a mixture of chloroform and alcohol. At the same time I would never unduly press forward bichloride of methylene, firstly because it is rather a difficult product to make, and, secondly, because it contains chlorine, which always has been, and is, a dangerous element. . . . You will gather from these observations that the temporary introduction of a member of the chlorine series into the anaesthetic series has been from the first a mistake — a mistake which must by necessity be met in the future by the exclusion of so objectionable an element."

Thus did Benjamin Ward Richardson simultaneously defend his bichloride of methylene against its detractors and criticise, if not damn, it himself. He was in a better position than most to do so having tried, over the years, more than 35 substances as anaesthetics. On this occasion his remarks

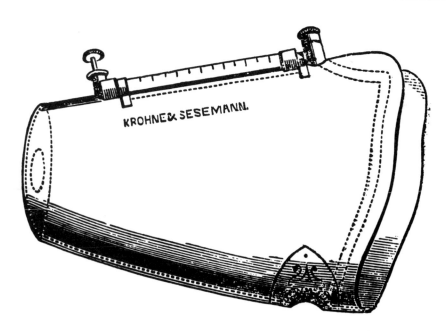

FIGURE 56

The inhaler described in the *Medical Times and Gazette* of November 23rd, 1872 by Benjamin Ward Richardson for "Methylene ether" which is what he called a mixture of methylene bichloride and ethyl ether and which, he believed, "stands hardly second to the safest anaesthetic I have ever experimented with — *viz.*, methylic ether gas".

were addressed, initially, to the Society of Anaesthetists. The title of his address was "The next great advance in Anaesthesia". Richardson considered that this would be the use of what he called methylic ether (the proper name for which is, nowadays, dimethyl ether, a gas with the formula $(CH_3)_2O$), a substance which he had discovered in 1867 and had used over 30 times to provide anaesthesia for surgical operations. Sir Benjamin Ward Richardson was an enthusiast and clearly his determination to introduce newer and safer anaesthetic agents had not diminished as the years had passed.

Such are the facts and opinions which I have been able to discover about Richardson's bichloride of methylene. "Bichloride of methylene" had a life, as an anaesthetic, of between 20 and 30 years. Whether it really was the compound Richardson thought it to be, and whether it really was safer than chloroform I cannot say. What is certain, however, is that "bichloride of methylene" worked and produced anaesthesia in several thousands of people.

For that, much thanks.

REFERENCES

[1] Spencer Wells, T. (1871) Bichloride of methylene (chloromethyl) in general surgery. Lancet, 2, 591–592.

[2] Anonymous (1867) Dr. Richardson on the bichloride of methylene as a general anaesthetic. British Medical Journal, 2, 345.

[3] Editorial (1867) Lancet, 2, 523–524.

[4] Anonymous (1868) Bichloride of methylene. British Medical Journal, 1, 407–408.

[5] Rendle, R. (1869) On the use of protoxide of nitrogen gas; and on a new mode of producing rapid anaesthesia with bichloride of methylene. British Medical Journal, 2, 412—413.

[6] Anonymous (1869) Death from bichloride of methylene. Medical Times and Gazette, 2, 466.

[7] Anonymous (1869) Death from bichloride of methylene. Medical Times and Gazette, 2, 524.

[8] Marshall, P. (1869) Death from bichloride of methylene. British Medical Journal, 2, 436.

[9] Anonymous (1869) Death from the administration of bichloride of methylene. Lancet, 2, 582–583.

[10] Richardson, B. W. (1869) On bichloride of methylene. British Medical Journal, 2, 487–488.

[11] Anonymous (1871) Death under the influence of methylene. British Medical Journal, 1, 456.

[12] Anonymous (1872) Death from bichloride of methylene at the Middlesex Hospital. British Medical Journal, 2, 417.

[13] Anonymous (1884) Death from bichloride of methylene. British Medical Journal, 2, 975–976.

[14] Anonymous (1884) Death from methylene. British Medical Journal, 2, 826.

[15] Spencer Wells, T. (1878) Lectures on the diagnosis and surgical treatment of abdominal tumours. British Medical Journal, 1, 925–928.

[16] Junker, F. (1883) Remarks on death from methylene and on the use of other anaesthetics. *British Medical Journal*, **2**, 104–107.

[17] Robbins, J. (1883) Bichloride of methylene. *British Medical Journal*, **2**, 271.

[18] Junker, F. E. (1868) New apparatus for the administration of narcotic vapours. *Medical Times and Gazette*, **1**, 171–173.

[19] Junker, F. E. (1867) Description of a new apparatus for administering narcotic vapours. *Medical Times and Gazette*, **2**, 590.

[20] Kirk, R. (1883) Remarks on bichloride of methylene. *British Medical Journal*, **2**, 1233–1234.

[21] Junker, F. E. (1884) Bichloride of methylene before the Academy of Medicine of Paris. *British Medical Journal*, **1**, 450–452.

[22] Spencer Wells, T. (1890) The Bradshaw Lecture on abdominal surgery. *British Medical Journal*, **2**, 1413–1416.

[23] Richardson, B. W. (1896) The next great advance in anaesthesia; including a new exposition of common insensibility. *Lancet*, **1**, 1047–1051.

An editorial footnote :—

Was "bichloride of methylene" really the substance which Benjamin Ward Richardson thought it to be? I asked Cyril Vesey, M.Sc., the Senior Biochemist in the Research Laboratory of the Department of Anaesthesia at St. Bartholomew's Hospital, London, to help unravel this chemical conundrum. I am most grateful for his work on the subject, of which the following is a summary.

It is unlikely that the chemical referred to as, *inter alia*, bichloride of methylene in this chapter was methylene dichloride, or dichloromethane, which is the present-day name for the compound which Richardson thought he had introuduced into anaesthetic practice in 1867. There is both chemical and clinical evidence to support this view. The chemical evidence is fourfold.

Firstly, the standard method of preparation at the time, used "nascent" hydrogen to replace one chlorine atom in each molecule of chloroform according to the equation

$$CHCl_2 + 2H^+ = CH_2Cl_2 + HCl$$

This was achieved by adding zinc to a mixture of chloroform and ethyl or methyl alcohol and then introducing small amounts of hydrochloric acid; on gentle warming, a liquid distilled over at $53\,^\circ C$. This was then fractionally distilled to produce a low yield of methylene dichloride.[1] The procedure described by both Benjamin Ward Richardson[2] and Robbins and Company[3] omitted the hydrochloric acid, and it is difficult to see how they could have produced methylene dichloride. Secondly, the boiling point of methylene dichloride is $40\,^\circ C$ whereas that of the product made by Robbins and Company was well above this at $53\,^\circ C$. At this temperature a mixture of substances with a constant boiling point was, presumably, obtained. The most likely possibility is a binary azeotrope, either of methylene dichloride and alcohol (boiling point $54 \cdot 6°C$, containing $88 \cdot 5$ per cent. by weight of methylene dichloride) or of chloroform and methyl alcohol (boiling point $53 \cdot 5°C$, containing $87 \cdot 5$ per cent. by weight of chloroform). Thirdly, independent chemical analyses at the time suggested that "methylene" was a mixture of chloroform and alcohol. Traub, whose results were quoted by Junker, in 1883, showed that one fifth of the product marketed by Robbins and Company was soluble in water[4], and this, together with its ready esterification to form a benzoate, shows that this fraction was, indeed, an alcohol. The remaining, water-insoluble fraction boiled at between $59°C$ and $60 \cdot 50°C$ (the boiling point of methylene dichloride is $40°C$ and that of chloroform is $61°C$), and its density was the same as that of chloroform at $1 \cdot 49$ (at $20°C$ methylene dichloride's is $1 \cdot 32$); it formed an isocyanide, which is a reaction characteristic of chloroform. It is interesting that, in theory, a mixture of one part (by volume) of methyl alcohol and four parts of chloroform has a density of $1 \cdot 35$, a figure which is virtually the same as that quoted for the anaesthetic agent known as "methylene", i.e. $1 \cdot 3495$ at $17°C$. M. Regnauld examined two different samples of "methylene" and found that they had a boiling point of $53°C$ and, on distillation, left a residue which, because of its odour and formation of a characteristic compound, he thought was methyl alcohol.[4] He also found that a mixture which was four parts of chloroform to one of methyl alcohol had a boiling point of $53°C$ and a density of $1 \cdot 363$ (that of pure methylene dichloride, at $15°C$ is $1 \cdot 335$, and the presence of methanol would decrease it), and found that when the methyl alcohol was removed from "methylene" by anhydrous calcium chloride that which remained was chloroform. Fourthly, the properties of "methylene" reported by Spencer Wells were not those of methylene dichloride. He stated that "methylene" was unstable and would keep for an hour only unless it contained some alcohol; he added that its vapour burnt.[5] Methylene dichloride is considered to be one of the most stable of the chlorinated hydrocarbons and does not burn.

The clinical evidence which suggests that "methylene" was not methylene dichloride is threefold. Firstly, the symptoms which preceded death during "methylene" anaesthesia[4] are similar to those now known to occur with chloroform. Most patients who died while under the influence of "methylene" were described as "livid" but, nowadays, we would expect deaths from methylene dichloride (a constituent of many modern paint removers) to be associated with signs of carbon monoxide poisoning. Inhalation of a mixture containing 690 parts per million of methylene dichloride for two hours gave rise to a carboxyhaemoglobin concentration of 6·2 per cent.[6] Anaesthetic concentrations of between 2 and 4 per cent. of "methylene" would have resulted in far higher levels of carboxyhaemoglobin. Secondly, Junker found that the mixture of four parts of chloroform to one part of methyl alcohol was very similar in its effects to "methylene", especially in the absence of vomiting which often accompanied the use of chloroform; he attributed this to the anti-emetic effects of methyl alcohol. Thirdly, chloroform, itself, was a most powerful agent the administration of which gave rise to a number of fatalities which were directly associated with the concentration inhaled by the patient. No doubt dilution of chloroform with methyl alcohol in the "methylene" reduced the concentration of chloroform, and, by allowing finer control, gave rise to fewer fatalities.

REFERENCES

[1] Greene, W. H. (1879) Sur le dioxyéthylméthylène et sur la préparation du chlorure de méthylène. *Comptes Rendus de l'Academie des Sciences*, **89**, 142–143.

[2] Richardson, B. W. (1896) The next great advance in anaesthesia; including a new exposition of common insensibility. *Lancet*, **1**, 1047–1051.

[3] Robbins, J. and Company. (1883) Bichloride of methylene. *British Medical Journal*, **2**, 271.

[4] Junker, F. E. (1884) Bichloride of methylene before the Academy of Medicine of Paris. *British Medical Journal*, **1**, 450–452.

[5] Spencer Wells, T. (1878) Lectures on the diagnosis and surgical treatment of abdominal tumours. *British Medical Journal*, **1**, 925–928.

[6] Ratney, R. S., Wegman, D. H., & Elkins, H. B. (1974) *In vivo* conversion of methylene chloride to carbon monoxide. *Archives of Environmental Health*, **28**, 223–226.

CHAPTER 14

NEW DRUGS AND STRANGE USES

As soon as ether and chloroform had established a foothold as anaesthetics, they began to be used for all sorts of other purposes and all kinds of treatment. For here were two new drugs of power, more definite and more dramatic in their action than the whole of the rest of the pharmacopoeia. In those days the pharmaceutical world was static, well-nigh permanently so, very unlike the present day when a never-ceasing flood of new and potent drugs pours forth from the synthetic chemists at such a rate that they do not always seem to have been fully considered and assessed.

Before the advent of ether the whole, united wisdom of the ages had produced little more than opium, mercury, quinine, digitalis, and a few purgatives. That was about the lot, so far as any definite action and real utility was concerned. The rest of the pharmacopoeia was a hotch-potch of traditional galenicals of uncertain composition and still more uncertain action — if, indeed, they had any action at all. Their main effects were, more often than not, as placebos.

So nobody really knew what these powerful newcomers were capable of doing. The only thing to do was to try them and find out.

It was early in January, 1847 that *The Lancet* published its first definitive account of the earliest use of ether anaesthesia in Great Britain,[1] and by the middle of that month was already advising caution in extending its use to the treatment of various medical conditions.

"Some have thought of its extension to medicine, and tetanus and hydrophobia have been mentioned as likely to be benefited by its use. Any such trials will assuredly end in disappointment, these diseases being diseases of motion, not of sensation."[2]

Sure enough, before the month was out, *The Lancet* published a letter from a somewhat crestfallen Dr. Ranking, of Bury St. Edmunds, who had tried ether in the treatment of tetanus.

"Having recently had a very severe case of tetanus under my care, I thought that I would give the ether a trial; I found, however, what a little reflection might have taught me, that it was even worse than useless, and that the spasms were fearfully augmented by every attempt at inhalation."[3]

Understandable, perhaps, with attempts at induction with crude ether alone, given by a man of the slightest experience — at this date no one had much practice at giving it. The fate of Dr. Ranking's patient is nowhere referred to.

Later in the same year *The Lancet* noted another attempt to use ether in the treatment of tetanus which had been first reported in the *Egyptian Spectator*. Dr. Franc, of the hospital at Caper-el-Hin, had administered ether by mouth — up to half an ounce at a time — for 28 days to a young man with severe tetanus "which had effected a cure".[4] Whether this was *post* or *propter*, who can say? Others tried it, unsuccessfully, as did Bransby Cooper at Guy's Hospital, London, whose efforts were to no avail since his young patient died of tetanus during a severe spasm 6 days after his first symptoms occurred.[5]

The following year it was chloroform's turn. From Birmingham came a report of a case, diagnosed as tetanus, which recovered, almost certainly fortuitously, after an inhalation of ether for a mere 45 minutes.[6] A patient who was unfortunate enough to have both hydrophobia and tetanus at the same time failed to recover. This is hardly surprising.

J. G. Lansdown, of Bristol, used ether in tetanus with good results.[7] He added that, since news of the discovery of ether anaesthesia had come to England some nine months earlier, he had used it on 242 occasions, 63 times in labour. Dr. Brickell, of New Orleans, gave (with other remedies) chloroform in mucilage by mouth and his patient with tetanus got better.[8] Dr. Frederick Gray, of Ottery St. Mary in Devon, the most persistent and patient of them all, gave chloroform inhalations to a ten-year-old boy with tetanus every two hours or so for a week, and used 3 lbs. of chloroform in all.[9] He, deservedly, had the satisfaction of seeing his young patient make a full recovery. I imagine that this case might hold the world record for the largest amount of chloroform given to a single patient. However, allowing for the age of the patient, Dr. Williamson, in Manchester, ran it pretty close. He gave chloroform to a six-week-old baby and kept it under, more or less, for 60 hours using 16 ounces in the process.[10] The infant recovered.

Anaesthetics were also used in the treatment of hydrophobia. Robert Allan, a surgeon stationed in Mauritius, described the case of Ramjan, an Indian servant-boy aged twelve, who was bitten by a mad dog in May, 1846.[11] A year later he developed hydrophobia. Ether inhalations controlled the spasms but Ramjan died. Dr. Allan proposed, in any future case, to begin with ether and follow it with alcohol intoxication for many hours "thereby giving time for the animal poison, if such there be, to work itself out of the system, if such a thing be possible". This rather resembles the agnostic's prayer "Oh God! If there is a God, save my soul, if I have a soul".

In 1848 a case, said to be of rabies, was successfully treated with chloroform by Dr. Ackerley, of Liverpool.[12] Abner H. Brown, of Lowell, Massachusetts, used a similar method in the treatment of a case of hydrophobia but his patient died.[13]

The next, non-surgical, use of anaesthetic agents was for the detection of malingering. As might be expected it was first used for this purpose in conscript armies. In April of 1847, Monsieur Baudens told the French Academy of Sciences of a soldier who had applied for discharge from the French army because of a spinal curvature.[14] The curvature disappeared under the influence of ether and "the deception the man practised was now clearly proved". Things worked the other way as well; a soldier with a stiff hip was suspected of malingering. He was given ether for twelve minutes until his muscles were relaxed and "then the reality of the disease was manifested". Monsieur Fix, a surgeon in the French army, thought up a scheme for distinguishing faked epilepsy from the real thing.[15] He said that in simulated epilepsy chloroform produced only its usual anaesthetic and relaxing effects, while in true epilepsy a fit could be induced at any time by chloroform; the administration of ether and chloroform simultaneously would, he said, augment the fit's duration and intensity. M. Fix suggested that this could be of medico-legal importance. However, these fallacies came to the notice of John Snow who, because of his own observations, was able to denounce the tests as completely unreliable saying ". . . if this assertion has been acted on, it must have led to great injustice . . ."[16] Hans Zocher, of Munsterlingen in Germany, reported the case of a pretended mute who tried to spend the winter in hospital because of his disability: a dose of chloroform betrayed his ability to speak. "His involuntary vociferation was of the most distinct and articulate character."[17] In 1870, a murderer in New York was suspected of feigning insanity. He was given chloroform and was questioned while he was recovering. He gave true and rational answers and when he realised what he had done he made a full confession.[18] This was one of the earliest uses of the "truth drug" so beloved by the daily press. G. K. Chesterton's Father Brown said the last word about truth drugs and lie detectors. Referring to a new machine for examining criminals a prison governor said "Now, in my opinion, that machine can't lie." "No machine can lie", replied Father Brown, "nor can it tell the truth."

A similar thing was reported in 1921.[19] In the United States a criminal accused of murder refused to speak for two weeks. He was given nitrous oxide and ether to the stage of excitement and, then, was able to talk. It is not stated what happened to him. Fifty years earlier, an American prisoner under sentence of death "was in such a state of wild excitement that no one dare enter his cell, and the sheriff called in the aid of a medical gentleman, who syringed chloroform upon the prisoner through the grating of the door until he was reduced to a state in which irons could be put upon him".[20]

Other curious uses of anaesthetics can, sometimes, be found. In 1855 an attempt was made to destroy an elephant with chloroform.[21] The animal, presumably a circus or zoo veteran, was 120 years old, had diseased feet and was unable to walk. A veterinary surgeon and a chemist, both from Birmingham, chloroformed it in ten minutes. They then gave it prussic acid and two doses of strychnine without effect. They continued the chloroform for three hours in the hope that this would kill the elephant, but it did not and the animal was allowed to recover. Finally the determined pair solved the problem by giving chloroform once more and then cutting a branch of the carotid artery. It is a pity that no doses are recorded. I would like to know how much chloroform an elephant could stand. I imagine that few people, even among veterinary surgeons, have tried to find out.

Descending from the sublime to the ridiculous, we next find chloroform recommended as an oyster opener.

"Chloroform is an excellent substitute for the oyster-knife. A little chloroform, it is said, applied to the shell, sends the dear little delicious creatures into a deep sleep, even though they be just out of their beds, and in the unconsciousness of their dreamhood, they gradually open and let in the enemy."[22]

In fairness to *The Lancet* it should be added that this tongue-in-cheek extract, entitled "Anaesthesia in Nutrition" was quoted from a Sheffield newspaper. It may be so, I don't like oysters, so I have never tried the method. Nor have I anaesthetised an elephant.

Another crazy method, which I do not intend to try, is the dropping of chloroform into the eye in an attempt to cure chronic inflammation of the lids with epiphora and intolerance to light. Amazingly enough, this was stated to give some relief.[23]

An attempted robbery with the aid of chloroform was briefly mentioned in 1850,[24] and the language used by *The Lancet* is worth quoting since it seems typical of the prose of the period as far as medical reporting is concerned.

"Both the *Kendal Mercury* and the *Carlisle Journal* contain an account of an attempt made, in Kendal, on Sunday week last, to rob an elderly clergyman, by the aid of chloroform. The clergyman, who was temporarily visiting the town, had taken up his residence at an hotel, to which the person charged with the nefarious act resorted, as is supposed, for its express purpose. The aged gentleman had retired to bed early on the night of the 13th. inst., and being unable to lock his door, had secured himself against intruders but inefficiently; he was subsequently awakened by the attempt of a person to render him powerless by placing a cloth over his mouth; and at the time of his rescue by those whom his cries brought to the apartment, a strong smell of chloroform is reported to have been perceptible, and two bottles of that substance are said to have been discovered. The matter will undergo investigation at the sessions. It is not the first time that an agent of good has been converted into an instrument of evil."

Another unfinished story about chloroform and crime, which first appeared in a London newspaper, was quoted by the *Boston Medical and Surgical Journal* in 1850.[25]

"Margaret Higgins and Elizabeth Smith, two women of depraved habits, were brought up to the Worship-Street Police Court for final examination, charged with having been concerned in administering chloroform to Mr. Frederick Hardy Jewitt, ... and subsequently robbing him of his watch, finger-ring, personal clothing, and various other articles. The prosecutor, who was unable to attend when the case was last before the magistrate, in consequence of severe illness resulting from the outrage to which he had been subjected, was now supported into court by his father, and accommodated with a seat in the counsel's box while his evidence was read over, ... but he evidently remained in such a shattered and debilitated condition that ... [he was allowed] ... to retire immediately he had attached his signature to his depositions."

Mr. Jewitt was a solicitor in London and I doubt that all his poor condition could be blamed on the chloroform itself: whether the women were convicted I have not been able to find out. There is an interesting sequel to this report. In 1851, the year of the Prince Consort's Great Exhibition at the Crystal Palace, John Snow wrote a letter to Lord Campbell[26] who was at the time advocating a "Prevention of Offences" Bill to the House of Lords. One clause of this Bill provided severe punishment for any attempt to administer chloroform, or any other stupefying drug, for unlawful purposes. Lord Campbell, Snow thought, was activated by the number of trials which had occurred at that time in which the defendant had been accused of using chloroform to further a crime. He may well have known of the clergyman's plight in Kendal and of the solicitor's entanglement with the two ladies in London. Snow considered that "the evidence against the prisoners, of attempting to produce insensibility by chloroform, was without any reason or possibility", and, being a lifetime abstainer from alcohol, had a further viewpoint.

"Knowing the weakness of human nature which leads a man, in the presence of all evidence, never to admit intoxication as possible in his own proper person,

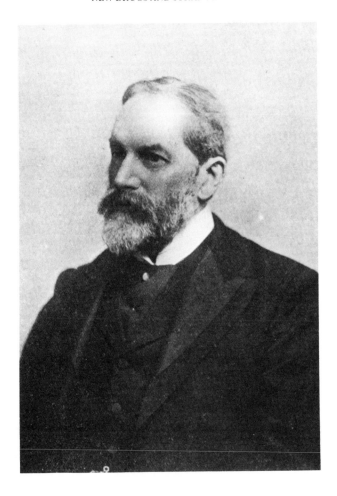

FIGURE 57

Dr. Ernest Sansom. 1838–1907. In 1865 he wrote *Chloroform: its action and administration.* He also wrote books on cardiology and antisepsis. He was the first to bring before the profession Pasteur's researches on fermentation. He was, also, a Consulting Physician to The London Hospital, Whitechapel.

CHLOROFORM:

ITS

ACTION AND ADMINISTRATION.

A HANDBOOK.

BY

ARTHUR ERNEST SANSOM, M.B. Lond.,

LATE HOUSE PHYSICIAN, AND PHYSICIAN-ACCOUCHEUR'S ASSISTANT TO KING'S COLLEGE HOSPITAL.

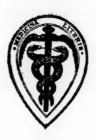

LONDON:

JOHN CHURCHILL AND SONS, NEW BURLINGTON STREET.

MDCCCLXV.

FIGURE 58
The title page of Sansom's book on chloroform.

Dr. Snow felt that, in any case where an intoxicated person had been robbed, such person might allege that he had been made insensible by narcotic vapour".

Lord Campbell did not agree with Snow's view and, after a while, agreed to differ. There the matter rested. Nonetheless, if John Snow thought the evidence was bad then it probably was.

Dr. Arthur Ernest Sansom gave evidence in a similar case in 1865 and pointed out that a period of at least five minutes was required to produce insensibility in a completely cooperative and prepared patient.[27] He was giving evidence in a case of a crime allegedly committed after a man had been rendered instantly unconscious by waving a handkerchief impregnated with chloroform under his nose.

Dr. Sansom was born in 1838, qualified in 1859 and, eventually became Physician to The London Hospital; he died on March 10th 1907. Sansom became very interested in anaesthesia during his early days and wrote an excellent book entitled *Chloroform: its action and administration* in 1865.[28] This was the year of the trial referred to. In his book he described his own inhaler for operations around the mouth. So he certainly knew something about his subject when he gave his evidence in court.

Chloroform was taken by mouth in certain cases — some of them suicidal and some with therapeutic intent. I came across ten cases of poisoning with chloroform taken in this fashion, six of which recovered after taking between 1 and 4 ounces of chloroform. The four deaths were caused by quantities varying from 1 to 6 ounces; the fatal dose appeared to vary considerably.

Chloroform was given for sea-sickness by Dr. William Henderson, of Perth in Scotland.[29] He stated that it would not prevent the initial sickness but, when the stomach was empty further sickness could be prevented by putting 10 to 15 drops of chloroform on to a piece of sugar which should then be sucked while sipping small amounts of cold water. Dr. Henderson said that this was a very successful remedy.

M. Dannecy, a pharmacien of Bordeaux, devised an elegant prescription for giving chloroform by mouth. This consisted of chloroform, oil of sweet almonds, gum arabic, syrup of orange flowers and distilled water.[30]

Dr. Heywood Smith, of St. Andrews, reported a rather remarkable journey made five years earlier in 1868.[31] He described this "Anaesthetic travelling" as follows:

"About five years ago I accompanied a patient of my father's, a highly nervous lady, to Boulogne, during nearly the whole of which journey she was under the influence of the tetrachloride of carbon. I commenced the administration in the

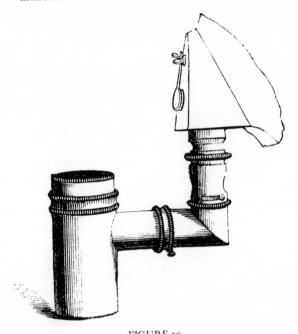

FIGURE 59

In his book Sansom again described his chloroform inhaler (it had first been described in the *British Medical Journal* on September 10th, 1864). It consisted of a cylinder (3″ long and 1½″ in diameter) lined with blotting paper or lint on which the chloroform was poured, and from which it vaporised. This shows how it was attached to a mask for use in the sitting position.

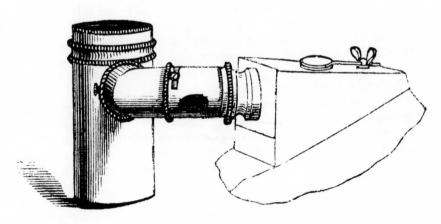

FIGURE 60

Sansom's inhaler adapted for use in the recumbent patient.

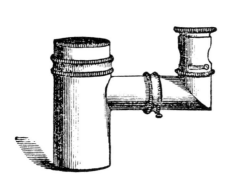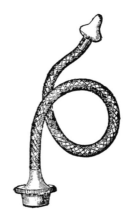

FIGURE 61
Sansom's inhaler with its adapter for nasal administration.

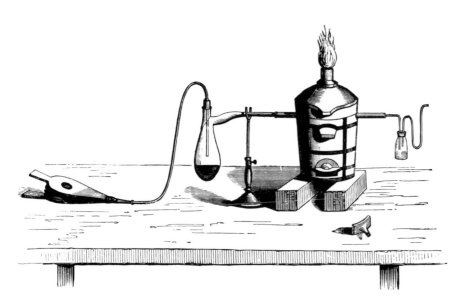

FIGURE 62
Duroy's method for the detection and estimation of chloroform. A retort with two
tubes is attached to a porcelain tube which passes through a charcoal furnace and ends
in a glass tube which dips into a vessel containing silver nitrate solution.

Chloroform, if present, is decomposed in the heated porcelain tube to produce
hydrochloric acid, which forms a white precipitate in the silver nitrate solution, the
residue of which is analysed volumetrically.

This illustration was included by Dr. Sansom in his excellent book.

177

railway, intermitted it during the change on to the steamer, kept it up during the passage, which entirely prevented any sea-sickness, and the patient did not recover consciousness until she was in her bed at Boulogne. Five or six weeks afterwards I went over to Boulogne and brought her back the whole way under the same anaesthetic, to her manifest great advantage. I can, therefore, confidently recommend anaesthesia, both as a means of conveying hyperaesthetic patients in their journeys, and also as a preventive of seasickness. I also think that the tetrachloride of carbon is a better agent for such work than chloroform, as it is less depressing, and requires a less quantity to produce the same effect, which is a point to be considered in a prolonged administration."

With the march of civilisation came bigger and better wars, and anaesthesia was used in the treatment of certain psychiatric conditions which, at the time, were called "shell-shock". I am sure that psychiatrists must have a much longer and more learned name for it now. While stationed at Taplow in Buckinghamshire during 1915 Major A. P. Procter, of the Canadian Army Medical Corps, reported three cases in which aphasia due to nearby shell explosions had been cured.[32] The first patient, who had been shelled at Ypres, remained aphasic for some weeks until he "was allowed to visit the village with some of his companions and while there became intoxicated. In this condition he 'found his voice' and for two days talked and sang incessantly". Two further cases were cured by ether anaesthesia; during the stage of excitement both soldiers were induced to speak. Sir William Osler had seen these patients with Major Procter and was so impressed that he wrote recommending the method for a similar patient he had seen at the American Hospital in Paignton, Devon who was, thereupon, cured by ether.

I came across nine instances of people found dead whilst inhaling anaesthetics. Indeed, the second death under anaesthesia ever reported was one of them. On February 8th 1848, eleven days after Hannah Greener had died under chloroform at Winlaton, a druggist's 17-year-old apprentice was found dead.[33] He had acquired the chloroform habit and inhaled it daily. At the time of his death the only other person in the shop was a boy of 12. Apparently, the apprentice had poured the chloroform on to a towel and inhaled it while leaning over the counter, and he had then fallen forward burying his face in the towel. Dr. Jamieson, one of several medical men summoned to the druggist's shop, performed artificial ventilation having intubated the trachea through the mouth: this is a very early example of this manoeuvre. Later a tracheostomy was performed but all attempts to revive the lad were to no avail.

Princess von Windischgrätz, who lived in Vienna and was a member of

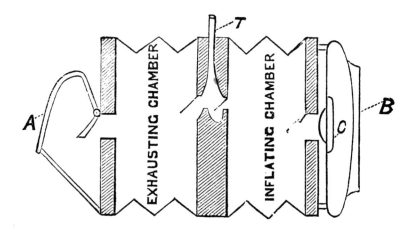

FIGURE 63

Dr. Sansom stressed the importance of having apparatus to hand for resuscitation during anaesthesia. The means of artificial ventilation which he preferred was the bellows, illustrated here, invented by Mr. W. Spencer Watson. The outlet was designed to be attached to two tubes which were inserted into the patient's nostrils, or to a single tube attached to a tracheostomy.

one of Austria's, then, leading families, was found dead after the self-administration of chloroform for headaches.[34] *The Lancet* wrote:

"If this accident were solitary and unprecedented, or if the fatal custom in which it originated was peculiar to the Princess Windischgrätz, no other comment would be needed other than a simple expression of regret that a mishap so lamentable should have occurred through a striking act of incautiousness. But the anodyne powers of chloroform have so wide and so justly-earned a reputation, and the pocket-handkerchief school of administrators has disseminated so general and reprehensible a carelessness in the inhalation of chloroform, that hundreds of persons still retain the impression that they may safely and easily lull the pain of neuralgia or any other acute disease by inhalation of the fumes of chloroform upon a handkerchief. It is a fact that many ladies are in the habit of alleviating their headaches by such means; that many others seek in chloroform, so employed, a remedy for facial neuralgia and periodic toothache. It is also a fact that the Princess Windischgrätz is only one of several who have fallen victims to their incautiousness . . ."

Joseph Toynbee, who was a Fellow of the Royal Society, and first aural surgeon to St. Mary's Hospital, London, was found dead on a couch in his consulting room on the 8th July, 1866.[35] He had been, apparently, experimenting on himself with chloroform and prussic acid in the treatment of tinnitus antrum. His watch and a paper on the effects of chloroform used for singing in the ears were found on a chair nearby. Toynbee had been inhaling chloroform from a cotton wool pad which still covered his mouth and nose when his body was discovered. He had, earlier, considered using Clover's apparatus but thought it too complicated for his purpose. He was, apparently trying Valsalva's method of inflating the Eustachian tube.

In 1903, Dr. E. Percy Court, of Hambledon in Hampshire, reported another case in which the chloroform habit had ended fatally.[36] A sick, nervous and, reportedly, hysterical woman of 42 had been bedridden for 18 years, and had, for a considerable time, inhaled chloroform each night to cure her insomnia. Initially this had been prescribed by her doctor. Later, she was found dead in her bed; the room smelled of chloroform and, by her bed, were an unstoppered bottle containing the drug and the handkerchief from which she usually inhaled the chloroform. She used an ounce of chloroform which cost fourpence, once or twice a day. As she was a pauper it is not easy to say where she got the money for this. Outdoor relief was not on a generous scale in those days.

Nitrous oxide also claimed its share of victims. In 1893, Dr. Gage Brown was called to see a 40-year-old London dentist who had been found dead in his surgery.[37] He found him still sitting in a chair opposite his gas apparatus, with the face mask still applied and his head having fallen on to his knees. One cylinder of nitrous oxide was turned on, but empty. A similar happening was reported in 1920 by Drs. James Holmes and Hedley Visick of Hampstead General Hospital in London.[38] Dr. Holmes had called at a practice to give a dental anaesthetic and had found the dentist dead in his operating chair. The mask was still pressed to the face, the dentist's head having fallen sideways over the arm of the chair on to the gas stand. The nitrous oxide cylinder was still supplying gas.

S. R. Wilson, a well-known Manchester anaesthetist, died on September 12th, 1927, during the self-administration of nitrous oxide and oxygen. His death was due to the premature exhaustion of an oxygen cylinder during an experiment he was making on himself.[39] Sidney Rawson was very interested in hypnotism, amongst other things. I myself saw dental extractions under hypnosis at a demonstration given by him. He may well have been using nitrous oxide to learn whether or not it increased susceptibility to hypnotism or suggestion. I am certain that there was no question whatsoever of his suicide. Only the year before he had been interested in ether convulsions, which problem had only just arisen, especially in Manchester where many of the early cases occurred. I am sure that the interest of this, to an anaesthetist of his originality and calibre,

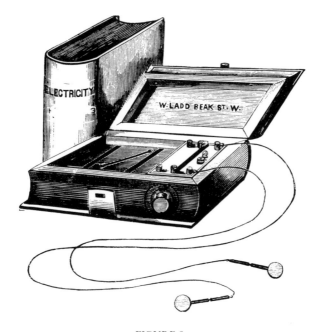

FIGURE 64

Sansom also thought that galvanism of the phrenic nerves would be useful. This is Dubois-Raymond's galvanic apparatus, the electrodes of which could be applied to the phrenic nerves either trans-cutaneously or, after dissection, to the exposed nerves themselves. Sansom's apparatus was disguised as a book entitled *Electricity*.

would preclude any thought of self-destruction. Incidentally, in 1921 he had collaborated with Dr. Kenneth Pinson in the production of the "Pinson Bomb" for ether anaesthesia.[40]

The uses of anaesthetics in general medicine were varied and widespread. References would be wearisome and pointless. Suffice it to record that, in the period following their introduction as anaesthetics, ether and chloroform were used in the following conditions at the dates mentioned.

Asthma	1847
Hysteria	1847
Insanity	1847
Laryngysmus stridulus	1847
Renal colic	1847
Whooping cough	1847

Chorea	1848
Delirium tremens	1848
Dysmenorrhoea	1848
Infantile convulsions	1848
Puerperal convulsions	1848
Strangulated hernia	1848
Typhus	1848
Strychnine poisoning	1850
Pulmonary consumption	1851
Lead colic	1852
Phagadaenic ulcers	1853
Retention of urine	1855
Stramonium poisoning	1881

Cholera, perhaps because it was so rapidly fatal and so resistant to all attempts at cure, was thought to be amenable to treatment with the new drugs quite early on. In 1846, even before the news of ether anaesthesia had arrived in Britain, it was suggested that nitrous oxide

"so far as I am aware, has not yet been tried in this disease; and yet, from its effects, we might expect to derive some benefit from its employment, as it would tend to restore the balance of the circulation, and relieve the congestion of the internal organs."[41]

Thus wrote Dr. T. Moore. Almost 40 years later, in 1885, rectal ether was used in 15 cases of cholera "in the hope of destroying the vitality of the cholera bacillus".[42] Well, it was worth trying, I suppose.

The inevitable Benjamin Ward Richardson, that Pooh Bah of Medicine, pops up in this chapter as he does in many of the others. He proposed the use of anaesthesia for animals prior to their slaughter.[43] For this purpose he advocated coal gas bubbled through bichloride of methylene, and had even gone so far as to design an apparatus for this,

"... consisting of a tin reservoir, made to hang on a nail in the wall of the slaughter-house, and intended to contain the bichloride of methylene. To this reservoir two india-rubber tubes were attached, one to be connected with a common gas-jet, the other terminating in a tin funnel, large enough to receive the nose of a sheep, and furnished with a strap and buckle, like those of a muzzle, for fixing it on the head. The muzzle being placed, the tap of the gas was to be turned, and the gas suffered to bubble through the bichloride, and to pass on to be breathed by the animal. In a minute, perfect insensibility to pain would be produced; and the animals were found to breathe the gas quietly, without struggling or apparent dread. For large slaughter-houses Dr. Richardson had designed a sort of passage, divided into chambers by doors which would open to admit an advancing truck, and would close as it passed through. The central chamber would be filled by the mixed vapour, and mere passage through it would render the animal insensitive to the knife, which would await its exit."

Why he added the bichloride of methylene is not easy to understand; the coal gas alone would have been just as effective, and much cheaper. After the meeting, (strangely enough Richardson had presented his idea to the Medical Society, in London), the audience sampled meat from a fowl slaughtered under this form of "anaesthesia", and found it untainted. *The Lancet* commended the method, hoped that it would be taken up by the Society for the Prevention of Cruelty to Animals, and suggested

"A few premiums or medals to slaughterers, for the skilful and effectual use of an anaesthetic, would probably do more to promote the objects of the Society than their whole machinery of penalties and informers."

This leads, without much ado, to a use of ether, (as a stimulant and antidote to chloroform), drawn from the pages of fiction and penned by no less an author than Sir Arthur Conan Doyle. One of the Sherlock Holmes short stories told in *His Last Bow* and published in 1917 tells of "The Disappearance of Lady Frances Carfax". She was a lonely, wealthy spinster abducted by a couple intent on robbing her of some jewels. Then, unable to murder her in cold blood, they decided to chloroform her and place her in a seemingly innocuous coffin to suffocate and be buried. At the very last moment this crime was thwarted by Holmes who, with Watson, forced open the coffin in which the body of Lady Frances Carfax lay, its head wreathed in cotton-wool soaked in chloroform. Holmes feared that she was dead and that they were too late to save her.

"For half an hour it seemed that we were. What with actual suffocation, and what with the poisonous fumes of the chloroform, the Lady Frances seemed to have passed the last point of recall. And then, at last, with artificial respiration, with injected ether, with every device that science could suggest, some flutter of life, some quiver of the eyelids, some dimming of a mirror, spoke of the slowly returning life."[44]

REFERENCES

[1] Boott, F. (1847) Surgical operations performed during insensibility. *Lancet*, 1, 5–8.
[2] Editorial (1847) *Lancet*, 1, 74–75.
[3] Ranking, W. H. (1847) Etherization in Tetanus. *Lancet*, 1, 135.
[4] Anonymous (1847) Ether in Tetanus. *Lancet*, 2, 139.
[5] Anonymous (1847) The Employment of ether in Tetanus. *Lancet*, 2, 313.

6 Baker, R. L. (1848) Instance of Tetanus successfully treated by Chloroform. *Lancet*, **1**, 610.

7 Lansdown, J. G. (1848) Hospital Reports. *Lancet*, **2**, 309–310.

8 Brickell, D. W. (1849) Case of traumatic Tetanus. *Boston Medical and Surgical Journal*, **40**, 122–123.

9 Gray, F. A. (1880) Traumatic Tetanus treated by chloroform inhalation; recovery. *Lancet*, **2**, 171.

10 Williamson, W. C. On the use of chloroform in a case of infantile convulsions. *Lancet*, **1**, 535.

11 Allan, R. (1847) Spasms of hydrophobia temporarily relieved by the inhalation of the vapour of sulphuric ether. *Lancet*, **2**, 409–410.

12 Ackerley, R. Y. (1848) Case of hydrophobic mania successfully treated with chloroform. *Lancet*, **2**, 122–123.

13 Brown, A. H. (1849) Case of hydrophobia. *Boston Medical and Surgical Journal*, **39**, 532–533.

14 Anonymous (1847) Practical application of Ether to Medical Jurisprudence, to distinguish feigned from real disease. *Lancet*, **1**, 411.

15 Anonymous (1848) Chloroform a test of Simulated Disease. *Lancet*, **1**, 288.

16 Snow, J. (1858) *On chloroform and other anaesthetics: their action and administration.* London: Churchill.

17 Anonymous (1858) A novel application of chloroform. *Lancet*, **1**, 305.

18 Anonymous (1870) Chloroform in criminal cases. *Lancet*, **1**, 445.

19 Anonymous (1921) Anaesthetics for an unusual purpose. *Lancet*, **1**, 819.

20 Anonymous (1866) *Lancet*, **1**, 639.

21 Anonymous (1855) Chloroforming an elephant. *Lancet*, **2**, 82.

22 Anonymous (1848) Anaesthesia in nutrition. *Lancet*, **1**, 111.

23 Anonymous (1850) On the use of Chloroform in Ophthalmia. *Lancet*, **1**, 85.

24 Anonymous (1850) Attempted daring robbery by the aid of Chloroform. *Lancet*, **2**, 490–491.

25 Anonymous (1850) Chloroform and Crime. *Boston Medical and Surgical Journal*, **42**, 104–105.

26 Snow, J. (1858) *On chloroform and other anaesthetics: their action and administration.* London: Churchill.

27 Anonymous (1865) Chloroform amongst thieves. *Lancet*, **2**, 490–491.

28 Sansom, A. E. (1865) *Chloroform: its action and administration.* London: Churchill.

29 Henderson, W. (1857) Chloroform in Sea-Sickness. *Lancet*, **2**, 103.

30 Anonymous (1855) Formula for the internal use of chloroform. *Lancet*, **1**, 462.

31 Smith, H. (1873) Anaesthetic travelling. *Lancet*, **2**, 355.

32 Procter, A. P. (1915) Three cases of concussion aphasia: treatment by general anaesthesia. *Lancet*, **2**, 977.

33 Anonymous (1848) Another death from chloroform. *Lancet*, **1**, 218.

34 Anonymous (1859) A fatal headache. *Lancet*, **1**, 351.

35 Obituary (1866) *Lancet*, **2**, 54.

36 Court, E. P. (1903) The chloroform habit acquired by a hysterical woman resulting in death. *Lancet*, **2**, 154.

37 Anonymous (1893) *Lancet*, **1**, 1319–1320.

38 Holmes, J. D., Visick, H. D. (1920) The danger of self administration of nitrous oxide gas. *Lancet*, **2**, 1167.

39 Obituary (1927) *Lancet*, **2**, 681.

40 Wilson, S. R., Pinson, K. B. (1921) A warm ether bomb. *Lancet*, **1**, 336.

41 Moore, T. (1846) Cholera. *Lancet*, **2**, 429.

42 Anonymous (1885) Rectal etherisation for cholera. *Lancet*, **2**, 588.

43 Anonymous (1871) Slaughtering under anaesthesia. *Lancet*, **2**, 616.

44 Conan Doyle, Sir A. (1917) *His Last Bow.* London: Murray.

CHAPTER 15

PROFESSOR SYME'S LECTURE ON
CHLOROFORM — AGAIN

James Syme, Professor of Clinical Surgery at Edinburgh, delivered his oft-quoted and famous (or notorious) address on chloroform anaesthesia to his students during the winter session of 1854–1855.[1] He did so during the third lecture of a course of 22, all of which were published in *The Lancet*.[2] Syme's remarks about chloroform, which must have taken no longer than ten minutes to deliver, were sandwiched between some comments about a court case in which he had been involved and his views on fistula-in-ano.

I have discussed Syme's lecture on chloroform in a previous essay[3] and, there, quoted the text in full. I make no apology for quoting it word for word once again, this time as a preface to the chapters on Edward Lawrie, and the Hyderabad Chloroform Commission. It was the cornerstone of Lawrie's thinking, and all his arguments, views and actions during this part of the chloroform controversy stemmed from Syme's teaching and, albeit limited, anaesthetic experience.

Syme delivered his lecture in the operating theatre of the Old Surgical Hospital at Edinburgh. At the time Edward Lawrie was just eight years old.

Professor Syme's lecture was as follows.

"I have now to speak of some cases in which chloroform will be given as usual, in consequence of the pain otherwise attendant on the operations to be performed; but before the patients are brought in I may take this opportunity of saying a few words regarding the use of chloroform, as you see that fatal cases, I am sorry to say, still occur, and that the medical journals, consequently, express doubts as to the use of chloroform at all, or say that, if used, it must be only with the greatest caution. Chloroform is no doubt a very powerful agent, sufficient to destroy the strongest individual if employed freely enough. Its fatal effects were shown at an early period in the following way: a lecturer in London was illustrating its action upon a guinea pig, which was placed in a glass jar along with some of the anaesthetic: the professor, in the eagerness of his discourse, left the animal too long under the jar, and it died. He explained to his audience the cause of the accident, but though the reasons he gave were satisfactory, yet an impression was made upon the public which was not soon effaced. In this respect, however, there is nothing peculiar to chloroform as a medicinal agent; opium, prussic acid, strychnia, &c., not only may, but often do destroy life, through being used in overdoses. But the question is, may it be used, judiciously, so as to do the good without exposing the patient to the risk of the evil? It is said in London that it cannot; that its risk is so great that it is only justifiable to use it in case of operations accompanied with an extreme degree of pain, or where stillness on the part of the patient is essential to success, and that the greatest caution is required in its administration; here we say that, if used with moderate care, it is perfectly safe. It was in this theatre that chloroform was first administered in public, by Dr. Simpson, seven years ago; since then it has been almost daily given here, yet we have not had a fatal case. It is true that one solitary instance of death from chloroform has occurred in another part of the hospital, but that case has nothing to do with us; so far as my department is concerned, it might as well have been at Guy's Hospital, or in Kamschatka, or anywhere else; indeed, it so happened, that at the very time when that unfortunate event was taking place in another part of the establishment, I was myself performing an operation on a patient under chloroform in this theatre.

"In inquiring into the reason of this difference between the experience of chloroform in London and here, we have not far to search for the explanation: it must lie in one of three things — viz, difference in the chloroform, difference in the patients, or difference in the mode of administration: with regard to the chloroform, I believe that most of that which is used in London is made in Edinburgh, and I know that some of the fatal cases might be shown to have occurred with Edinburgh chloroform.

"With respect to the patients, it appears that great care is taken in London to use chloroform only in persons free from chest affections, especially cardiac derangements: here we never ask any questions as to the state of the heart or constitution of the patients. In all cases where chloroform is required for an operation, it is freely given. Now, considering the frequency of cardiac disease, and particularly of fatty heart, — which, in fact, is I believe rarely absent, at any rate in elderly persons, — and considering also the immense number of patients operated on, you cannot doubt that many hundreds with fatty degeneration of the heart have had chloroform administered to them here; we even give chloroform without scruple, where we know disease of the heart exists. Within the last week, a case in point occurred in my own practice. A patient, with great dread of pain, and also with a horror of chloroform, had long endured severe pain from his disease, till existence had become a burden, because he could not venture to undergo the necessary operation without chloroform, while his medical adviser considered that to take it would be for him almost certain death, on account of organic disease known to exist in the heart; for which he had consulted, and which it may be remarked had been recognised by, Dr. Addison, of Guy's Hospital. At length his medical attendant said to him, that he had suffered so much from his complaint, that even if he died under chloroform this would be better than remaining as he was; while, if it should so happen that he should recover, he would be able to enjoy the rest of his life free from the disease. The patient could not resist the force of this argument, and came to Edinburgh prepared for either alternative. I performed the operation under chloroform; and the first thing he did on waking was to ask for a cigar.

"As another example, I may mention the case of an old gentleman, aged seventy-four, affected with disease of the heart, from whose bladder I removed a

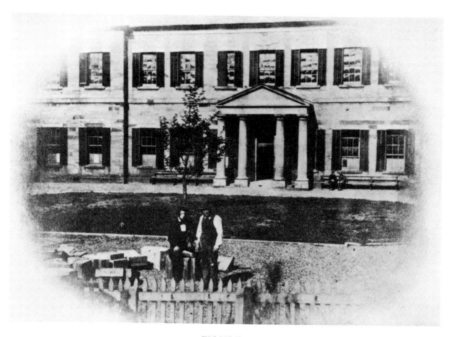

FIGURE 65
The Old Surgical Hospital, Edinburgh, in 1853. It was in this building, which still stands, that Professor Syme delivered his lecture which dealt with chloroform anaesthesia. One of the men in the foreground is "John", who was the surgical porter at the time.

large stone, some years ago. Chloroform was administered as he lay in bed; and he was put so fully under its influence, that he was taken from the bed, was operated on, and put back to bed, before he woke from his sleep. He recovered perfectly; but some time afterwards died, and Dr. Begbie, on examining the body, found the disease of the heart, which had been diagnosed during life. We cannot, therefore, attribute the absence of deaths here to our being more discriminating than others in the patients to whom we administer chloroform; the very reverse, in fact, being the case.

"I think then, gentlemen, that we are necessarily led to the conclusion, that the difference of results depends on difference in the mode of administration. We know that in other cases differences in the method of procedure have led to differences of results — e.g., it was said in London, that amputation at the ankle invariably caused sloughing; but it turned out that the surgeon who made this statement, performed the operation in a manner that deviated much from the principles on which it is here performed successfully, and which led inevitably to sloughing. So of dividing stricture by external incision, it was said that extravasation of urine must necessarily take place in a dangerous manner, and that other serious complications may occur; but it turned out that the incision had been made without guide on a silver catheter — in short, with such deviations from principles as fully to account for the results.

"So far as I can ascertain, from what I have heard and read upon the subject, there are important differences between the mode of administration of chloroform here and in London. It appears that here it is given according to principle, there according to rule. There great attention is paid to the number of drachms or minims employed; here we are entirely regardless of the amount used, and are guided only by the symptoms of the patient. The points that we consider of the greatest importance in the administration of chloroform are — first, a free admixture of air with the vapour of the chloroform, to ensure which, a soft porous material, such as a folded towel or handkerchief is employed, presenting a pretty large surface, instead of a small piece of lint, or any other apparatus held to the nose. Secondly, if this is attended to, the more rapidly the chloroform is given the better, till the effect is produced; and hence, we do not stint the quantity of chloroform. Then — and this is a most important point — we are guided as to the effect, not by the circulation, but entirely by the respiration; you never see anybody here with his finger on the pulse while chloroform is given. So soon as breathing becomes stertorous we cease the administration; from what I have learned, it is sometimes pushed further elsewhere, but this we consider in the highest degree dangerous. Attention to the tongue is another point which we find of great consequence. When respiration becomes difficult, or ceases, we open the mouth, seize the tip of the tongue with artery forceps, and pull it well forward; and there can be little doubt that death would have occurred in some cases if it had not been for the use of this expedient. We also always give the chloroform in the horizontal position, and take care that there is no article of clothing constricting the neck.

There are thus considerable differences between our practice and that which prevails more or less elsewhere. We use no apparatus whatever, take the respiration for our guide, attend to the condition of the tongue, and never continue beyond the point when the patient is fully under the influence of the anaesthetic.

"You observe that in this matter I am very far from taking any credit to myself; all that I have done is to follow the example of Dr. Simpson, and all that I would say respecting our brethren in London, is that they have not been so fortunate as to get into the right way in the first instance, and I would urge upon them to banish all previous notions, and to keep in view the essential points to which I have alluded; then, if unfortunately there should still be fatal cases, I shall not presume to speak further upon the subject. As the matter at present stands, the discussions prevalent in the profession tend to give the public a dread of chloroform, and to limit the advantages which it confers; and so long as the difference of opinion seemed due to important difference of practice, I felt called upon to address to you the observations I have made."

REFERENCES

[1] Syme, J. (1855) Lectures on Clinical Surgery delivered during the winter session of 1854–5. *Lancet*, **1**, 55–57.
[2] Index. (1855) *Lancet*, **1**, 665.
[3] Sykes, W. S. (1960) *Essays on the First Hundred Years of Anaesthesia. Volume I.* Edinburgh: Livingstone.

CHAPTER 16

HYDERABAD

We know much of the scientific controversy which, focused on Hyderabad, raged around the world. It would be interesting, perhaps, to have a glimpse of Hyderabad, and of Lawrie's working conditions and methods.

In 1895 "Medical Hyderabad" was described by a correspondent for the *British Medical Journal.*

"In the Nizam's domain of Hyderabad, in the Deccan, medical treatment and medical education have reached a high standard of excellence. Here was held the famous Chloroform Commission, which was due to the liberality and scientific interest of the Nizam and the energy and enthusiasm of Dr. Lawrie, the Presidency surgeon.

"The hospital, which stands in the centre of the picturesque city of Hyderabad, is small and ill-constructed; but still it answers its purpose very well, and perhaps in some ways suits the peculiar habits and customs of the people better than larger and more systemised institutions. A number of small apartments open on to a courtyard. In these women can live in 'purdah' or seclusion and according to their caste rules, or patients can be visited and waited upon by their relatives, which privilege induces them to go into hospital and be properly treated. There are also a number of small wards. Most of the cases treated are surgical. The operating theatre is open on all sides to the air, excepting that on which the students sit on rising tiers of seats. Chloroform is administered in a scientific and methodical manner, which may be copied with advantage in the London hospitals. The patient is laid on the table and stripped to the waist, Dr. Lawrie considering it more important to watch the respirations than the pulse. Each case is minutely recorded at the time, and all particulars as to the name and age of the patient and the nature of the case are entered in a book. The chloroformist calls out aloud to the clinical clerk standing at the head of the table with the record book in his hand minute by minute, indeed, second by second, the particulars as to the amount of chloroform administered, the respiration and pulse, etc. . . . Each senior student is taught in turn how to give chloroform, and holds the post of chloroformist for a month. Dr. Lawrie's large experience and careful and minute observations, extending over several years and including many thousands of cases, confirm him strongly in the opinion that the heart never becomes dangerously affected until after the breathing has stopped, and that, if chloroform is properly given, it has no injurious or dangerous effect upon the heart; in fact, all his experience confirms the view of Syme that we should be guilded as to the effect of chloroform, not by the circulation, but entirely by the respiration. . . . It is certain that in chloroform administration the pulse can only give secondhand information of something having gone wrong which might have been prevented by proper attention to the breathing. . . .

"The students of this interesting little medical school are Mohammedans, Hindus, Parsees, Eurasians and English. Five women are at present studying with the men, and are given the same opportunities of administering chloroform and performing operations as they. The latter seemed a special feature of this school, as Dr. Lawrie, heart and soul a surgeon and teacher, is anxious to turn out thoroughly well trained men and women surgeons from his school. He speaks very highly of the capacity of the native students and surgeons to perform the best work, and he shows no trace of that jealousy and suspicion of the native races which spoil some of the best work and teaching in India.

"With a hospital imperfectly constructed, and a school deficient in so many of the things which exist in the splendidly organised medical schools of Calcutta and Madras, Dr. Lawrie has by his enthusiasm and tact overcome all obstacles and has succeeded in creating a native medical school which gives no mean results in what was till recently the most retrograde of the native States of India. . . .

"The nursing arrangements are under the direction of Miss Lawrie, who, having received a thorough training as a nurse and sister in The London Hospital and the Children's Hospital, Chelsea, has successfully introduced the English nursing system, and has established a school where native nurses are trained both for hospital and private nursing.

"The hospital, the medical and nursing school are supported by the Nizam's Government."[1]

This is a very nice, and worthy tribute to Lawrie's enthusiasm, with which I thoroughly agree — with one exception. Tact is the very last word which could properly be applied to him!

Clarence Read also described what he saw in the course of a visit to Lawrie's hospital in 1894.

"During a recent visit to Hyderabad, Deccan, I had the pleasure of seeing chloroform administered on several occasions according to the method adopted by Surgeon-Lieutenant-Colonel Lawrie, the inhalations being conducted under his personal supervision. The routine of administration is briefly as follows: — The patient walks, if possible, or is carried into the operating theatre and lies down on the operating table with the chest uncovered. Four students then undertake the management of the patient. The first student announces so that everyone present may hear all the phenomena and the exact time of occurrence from the beginning of the administration until the patient recovers consciousness, the amount of chloroform given, the variations of pulse respiration, &c., all being noted. The second student writes down the same on specially arranged forms. The third student stands on the administrator's right with a drachm measure-glass and a bottle of chloroform, and measures it out as required. The fourth student is the administrator. He takes a cone of canvas, stiffened on either side with a thin piece

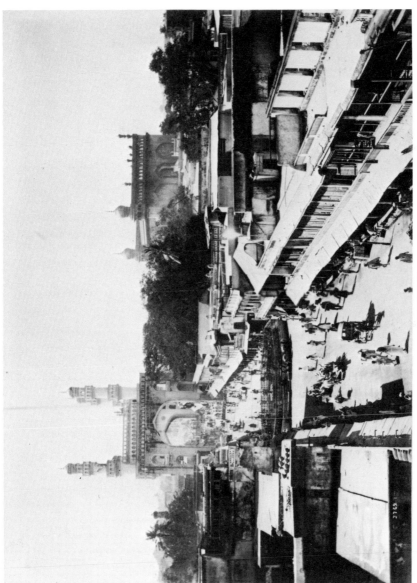

FIGURE 66

The main streat of Hyderabad in the central plateau of southern India in about 1890, showing the Charminah which was designed as the city's centrepiece. In 1890 the city of Hyderabad was the capital of the state of Hyderabad which was the largest princely state in India and was ruled over by the enormously wealthy Nizam who was the most powerful Muslim ruler in India. At that time the state of Hyderabad was independent, but was under British protection.

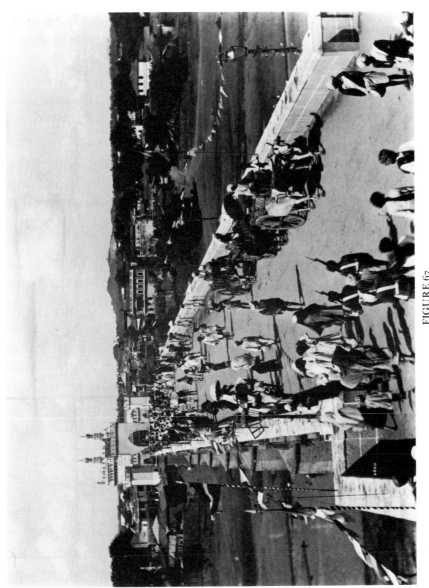

FIGURE 67

The entrance to the city of Hyderabad about 1890. The old, walled city and the parts outside the walls housed the wealthy and the desperately poor. The main British military settlement was a short distance away at Secunderabad. Hyderabad is now the capital of the state of Andrha Pradesh.

of cane. In the apex of the cone is placed a piece of clean cotton-wool, on which is poured one drachm of chloroform. The cone is then held over the nose and mouth, but not in close apposition. Drachm doses are poured on the wool every minute until struggling commences, the dose is then reduced to half a drachm every forty-five seconds. Anaesthesia being complete, the smallest amount possible to keep the patient under is administered. If signs of irregular breathing appear after the patient has become unconscious the inhalation of chloroform is withheld until it becomes regular, artificial respiration being performed if necessary. Respiration is what they look to as a warning of approaching danger, and not the pulse. Dr. Lawrie is present during the whole time, correcting any inaccuracies in recording phenomena. The patient is not removed from the operating table until he shows signs of return to consciousness."[2]

An earlier visitor to Hyderabad had also noticed the exceptional care with which Lawrie's pupils gave chloroform. M. G. Naidu wrote:

"The first things which strike a visitor to the Afzulgunj Hospital, Hyderabad, are the extraordinary care and skill with which chloroform is administered by the students of that institution to a large and indiscriminate number of patients. The administration of chloroform in Hyderabad appears to have been reduced to a fine art, and every additional case is a step towards the perfection of that art."[3]

Noticing the confidence which the students soon acquired with the giving of chloroform, Dr. Naidu remarked:

"Whence this confidence? Is it inborn? No, for many of the students at first hold the chloroform cap with trembling fingers. Is it the result of vast experience? No, for no student gets a chance of chloroforming the hospital patients for more than a month at a time. The origin of their confidence is rather to be found, in the first place, in the habit and as it were, the tradition of the school; and in the second place it is undoubtedly due to the immediate presence and personal teaching of Surgeon-Lieutenant-Colonel Lawrie, who holds himself, and not the students, responsible for everything which happens during an operation."

Lawrie's method, as detailed above, is then described in much the same detail, together with one interesting addition.

"Dr. Lawrie objects to the cap being kept on the face for even a second after the anaesthesia is complete, for the very palpable and sufficient reason that this is all the chloroformist has to produce and that anything beyond it is poisoning;... Dr. Lawrie, in common with other authorities, prescribes the abolition of the corneal reflex as the safest guide under ordinary circumstances to the establishment of complete anaesthesia."

Lawrie, as we know, was a most ardent and persuasive advocate of his method for giving chloroform which, in his hands or under his own supervision, worked extremely well. He, clearly, was a most persuasive host to those who came to see his hospital and study his methods.

In 1897, a short description of the town of Hyderabad was given in an article which described the outbreak of plague in Bombay and gave accounts of other towns to which the disease had spread. Hyderabad was once the principal town in Sind and, in 1891, had a population of 54,512; the birth-rate was 40 per 1,000, and the death-rate about 30 per 1,000. It was built on a limestone plateau three miles to the east of the Indus River.

"The bazaar is extensive, forming one street the entire length of the town, which is celebrated for its lacquered and ivory work, as well as silk embroidery.

The water supply is pumped from the Indus into settling tanks near the river bank, and after the greater part of the mud has subsided is distributed without filtration by means of cisterns and standpipes. There is no proper system of drainage; waste water stagnates in cesspools, percolates into the ground, or in some places is drained off in gutters to the lower quarters of the town."[4]

It is a little hard that Lawrie, after having lived in an insanitary place like this for sixteen years should die *of typhoid* in a health resort on the south coast of England!

REFERENCES

[1] Anonymous (1895) Medical Hyderabad. *British Medical Journal,* **1**, 989–990.
[2] Read, C. (1895) The Hyderabad method of administering chloroform. *Lancet,* **1**, 199.
[3] Naidu, M. G. (1893) The administration of chloroform in Hyderabad. *Lancet,* **2**, 365–366.
[4] Anonymous (1897) The Plague. Chronicle of the Epidemic. *British Medical Journal,* **1**, 937–939.

CHAPTER 17

EDWARD LAWRIE AND THE HYDERABAD
CHLOROFORM COMMISSION

Lieutenant-Colonel Edward Lawrie (1846–1915), of the Indian Medical Service, was Residency Surgeon at Hyderabad, in India, and was also a well-known figure in late-Victorian, medical journalism. He was, above all, a chloroform enthusiast — a fanatical, pugnacious and doctrinaire person who was not prone to let awkward or contrary facts upset or disturb his own theories and beliefs.

As far as Lawrie was concerned, he and his hero and former chief, Professor James Syme, were the only true believers. Syme was dead, and all others who remained were heretics. The whole rank and file of Medicine, except the Lieutenant-Colonel himself, seemed to be out of step. If only everyone could have accepted his advice and have used his methods there would never have been any more deaths from chloroform anaesthesia. It was, as far as Edward Lawrie was concerned, as simple as that.

Lawrie was a person with such an *idée fixe* that he was, naturally, a prolific writer in the journals of his day. After all, if one is the privileged and unique possessor of an absolute, infallible truth, it is a duty to share it with less-enlightened people, even if the disputed facts have to be beaten into their thick heads with the intellectual equivalent of a sledgehammer. Understandably, then, he tended to repeat himself. The more the opposition raged around him, the more he re-iterated his same, old arguments. Lawrie's letters, together with those of his opponents during the controversy (which went on for some 25 years) would fill a bulky volume of over a hundred thousand words — and this would not include those several, long reports which occupied no less than 350 columns of small print in the principal medical journals of the day. Clearly, any account of these events must rely on the strict editing of carefully chosen abstracts.

Without doubt, the controversial Edward Lawrie was an interesting man. In spite of all that his critics said, it must be admitted that he was, arguably, the most successful user of chloroform anaesthesia who ever lived. His own experience, amongst the vast population of India, was enormous and, as a result, his opinions are worthy of the most careful assessment. The work that he did, the views that he held and the influence that he had, all combine to make him far too interesting a person to be allowed to remain as a shadowy, half-forgotten figure.

It was not at all easy getting to know what the real Edward Lawrie was like but, eventually, and with a great deal of help from many people, I was able to correspond with his grand-daughter in Africa and, through her, to find and to talk to an elderly Scottish lady who had been a great friend of Lawrie and his wife.

Mrs. Armstrong, Lawrie's grand-daughter, had spent much of her childhood with him because her parents were for long periods away from home on foreign service. She was, obviously, extremely fond of her grandfather. She recalled that, soon after he had qualified from Edinburgh in 1867 he went off to China as a ship's surgeon; he was not at all a good sailor and, when called to a seasick patient, groaned and said, with his usual candour, "I am seasick too!"

Edward Lawrie was responsible for bringing up his younger brothers and sisters, which must have been a great strain — not least financially. He had a liking for horse-racing and bridge, both of which were expensive hobbies. On one occasion, he won a major part of the £75,000 prize on the Calcutta Sweepstake but, when he died, his widow was virtually penniless. He had been, I feel sure, far too honest to have taken advantage of his sixteen years' employment with the enormously wealthy Nizam, who was the hereditary ruler of the state of Hyderabad. No doubt, he could have feathered his nest, but I am certain that the idea never occurred to him. The Nizam's opinion of, and respect for, Lawrie may be judged from the fact that he awarded Mrs. Lawrie a pension of £600 a year following the death of her husband; this was no mean sum in those days.

Mrs. Armstrong recalled that her grandfather never seemed to be dull or bored; rather he was impetuous and had a zest for life. She remembered how, on one occasion, he got the entire household up at some unearthly hour to go and see either the first or the second aeroplane to fly across the English Channel. That would have been in 1909. While in China, he had acquired a passion for Pekinese dogs, and his grand-daugher had vivid memories of his holding court in his bedroom each morning, surrounded by his five Pekinese. To the best of Mrs. Armstrong's recollection Lawrie left his London home, at 115a, Harley Street, in 1908 or 1909. (A perusal of Kelly's Post Office directories reveals that he was last at the address in 1909.) She certainly remembered, however, giving chloroform for him when she was eight years old — yes, eight — during an emergency operation.

On leaving London Lawrie went to live at Hove in Sussex and, there, had two mentally ill patients under his care. One of them was a relative of the Nizam of Hyderabad. Later on, Lawrie moved to a house called "Westfield" where he lived until his death. The ostensible reason for this

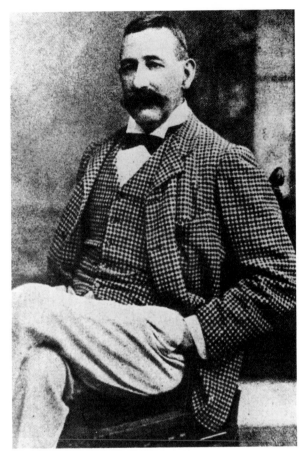

FIGURE 68

Edward Lawrie, I.M.S. 1846–1915. "One of the most influential participants in the frail history of Anaesthesia's first hundred years."

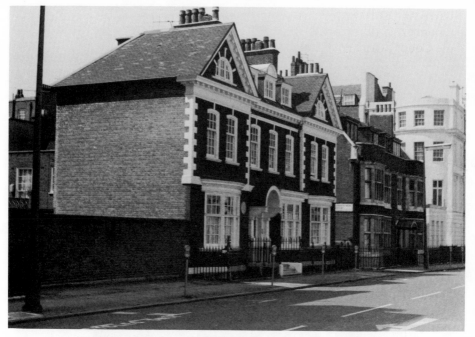

FIGURE 69

Edward Lawrie's London home, during the latter part of his life. From this address, 115a, Harley Street, London, he continued his campaign in support of the absolute safety of chloroform, based upon his own personal and amazing record. There is a "blue plaque" to the left of the front door; this refers, not to Lawrie, but to Sir Ernest Pinero, the playwright, who lived in the house immediately after Lawrie left to reside in Worthing.

move was to provide more room for his patients, but his grand-daughter thought that the real reason might have been that the new house overlooked the County Cricket Ground!

During these latter years, certainly up to the outbreak of the First World War, Edward Lawrie continued to write forceful, if not vitriolic, letters on his favourite topic — the safety of chloroform anaesthesia if properly administered. Near the end of his life he was able to emerge from the relative quietude of retirement and, despite ill-health, was once again to be of service to the Indians he knew so well. He must have been the sort of man to whom retirement and idleness was a terrible thing. Suddenly, two hospitals full of wounded, homesick Indian soldiers appeared on his very doorstep; for him, it must have seemed that life had begun again. Unfortunately, he did not enjoy this for more than about six months. Edward Lawrie died from typhoid on the 22nd August, 1915.

I met Mrs. Douglas, the elderly Scottish lady who knew Edward Lawrie and his wife well, in her lovely house overlooking Loch Tay in Perthshire. She remembered Lawrie as an energetic man who made swift, and generally wise, decisions. He held very decided opinions when he knew these were based on careful and, to him, convincing research. He was a hard worker, and was intolerant of slackness or mental laziness. He did not appear to be bitter, although he was a keen fighter for the principles in which he believed. He had a wide circle of friends, was debonair, hospitable, cheerful, gay, witty and much beloved by the young, whom he encouraged in work and in play. (This must have been so. He employed his grand-daughter as a chloroformist at the age of eight!) He was implacable in his opposition to those of his colleagues who disagreed with his carefully considered opinions. Admirably, he fought for what he really believed to be true — this, without question, is an excellent quality. Whether his beliefs were correct, or not, is another matter.

There we have the opinions of two people who knew Edward Lawrie well, and were devoted to him. As a private individual he must have been a very likeable man.

For more dispassionate accounts of his life we must look elsewhere. His obituaries in the *British Medical Journal*[1] and *The Lancet*[2] gave the salient features of his life.

Lawrie was born on May 17th, 1846 and educated at Edinburgh University (from where he qualified in 1867) and in Paris. He was Professor Syme's house surgeon at the Royal Infirmary in Edinburgh and then, following a controversial episode at the hospital, entered the Indian Medical Service in March 1872. He rose to the rank of Surgeon Lieutenant-Colonel before retiring from the Service in 1901. While in India he was for part of the time surgeon to the Medical College Hospital in Calcutta and also the College's Professor of Physiology. Thereafter, he became Professor of Surgery at the Lahore Medical College but he gave up this appointment in 1885 to become the Residency Surgeon at Hyderabad "the premier Indian native state, a post which is one of the most important medical appointments in India." As Residency Surgeon Lawrie

"was able to enlist the sympathies of the Nizam in the very interesting medical and physiological problems involved in the administration of chloroform. . . . it was at his suggestion that the Indian Chloroform Commission of 1889–90, of which His Highness the Nizam of Hyderabad paid the expenses, was appointed. He was best known . . . for his views on anaesthesia, being an ardent advocate of the claims of chloroform to be the best and safest anaesthetic for general use. His views on the subject were published in a book entitled *Chloroform: A Manual for Students and Practitioners* (1901)."

Lawrie retired from India in 1901, returned to Britain and practised as a consulting physician in London. He retired from this work in 1908–9 and went to live at Hove, in Sussex. At the outbreak of the First World War he was appointed to the staff of the Indian Hospital in Brighton (the Pavilion and the York Place Hospitals). This honour was not his for long; he died, on August 22nd, 1915 after a three month illness and was buried at Hove, with full military honours.

Sir Thomas Lauder Brunton, F.R.S. who was, at the time on the staff of St. Bartholomew's Hospital, London, added his own personal appreciations.

"The death of Colonel Edward Lawrie was to me a great shock . . . for he retained his appearance of youth and his energy to a much greater extent than most of his contemporaries, so that it seems almost impossible to believe that more than fifty years have passed since he and I used to walk in the early mornings to the botanical class in Edinburgh University. . . . While he was a student and house-surgeon in Edinburgh, Lawrie became thoroughly convinced that the view of his old teacher, Professor Syme, was correct and that chloroform only killed through the respiration and not through the heart. As many people, especially in this country, upheld the opposite view, Lawrie prevailed upon the Nizam to have a series of experiments instituted on monkeys to prove this point. Without exception these monkeys all died from failure of the respiration. As the result of these experiments did not meet with universal acceptation, Lawrie persuaded the Nizam to have a second Commission to investigate the action of chloroform, and to this . . . he invited . . . myself. Sometimes his zeal for truth caused him to see only one side of it and led him into polemics which would have been better avoided. Nevertheless, when all is said and done, Lawrie's virtues were many and his faults were few."[1, 3]

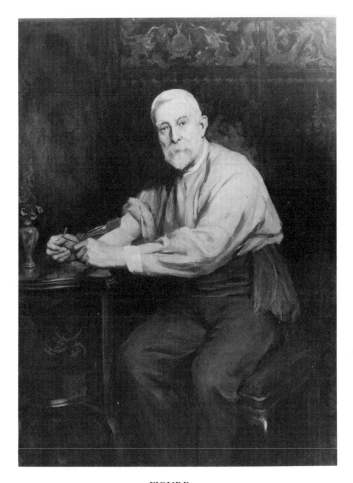

FIGURE 70

Sir Thomas Lauder Brunton 1844–1916.

Herkomer's portrait of Brunton which now hangs in the Great Hall of St. Bartholomew's Hospital, London. On his right arm is a Marey Sphygmograph for recording variations in the pulse wave of the radial artery. The vase contains a foxglove, from which digitalis is extracted.

Dr. Dudley Buxton, who had been one of the most active opponents of Lawrie's views wrote "Lawrie did much for the science of anaesthesia, and though we may not follow all his teaching we must recognise the value of his work, since it was he who stirred the water and many were healed."[4]

The Lancet, itself, felt that Lawrie's various obituaries had not given sufficient account of his efforts to discover the truth about chloroform anaesthesia, and published its own appraisal of his work, together with a summary of the controversy.

"Undoubtedly his work was excellent and will live after him, even though the dogmatic side of his teaching has been already toned down and his favourite theories have undergone material modification. Lawrie sought to prove the eternal verity, as it seemed to him, of Syme's somewhat truculent pronouncements on the action of chloroform; and though the disciple failed to accomplish his self-imposed task, nevertheless he achieved a great work — he compelled the profession to restudy the chloroform problem and to reconstruct the system by which that anaesthetic should be given. . . . That Lawrie should have been disappointed with the reception of the labours of himself and his co-workers was to be anticipated. His early association with Syme, a man of convincing personality, gave to Lawrie his faith, and to it he adhered until his death with something like a fanatic's tenacity. . . . For his enthusiasm, for his unconquerable efforts to try every means whereby the truth should be established, Lawrie earned perhaps insufficient praise. The Hyderabad Commissions and those subsidiary to them accumulated a vast amount of knowledge, and this has influenced both the science and the practice of anaesthesia. . . . A study of Snow's closely reasoned pages shows that he appreciated the fallacies of Syme and his school, and, indeed, Snow's very words can be quoted to disprove many contentions advanced by Lawrie and his fellow-workers. Yet to Lawrie we owe a debt of gratitude since his investigations gave us light, while his enthusiasm and dogged perseverance heartened other workers. Though such labours may bring neither honour nor advancement, they tend ever towards the revelation of truth."[5]

Surgeon-Major Lawrie, as he then was, fired the first broadside in his long campaign in January, 1889. This was at the prize-giving ceremony for the students at the Hyderabad Medical School, of which Lawrie was the Principal. The guests of honour were Their Royal Highnesses the Duke and Duchess of Connaught. Lawrie delivered a short speech, the substance of which was reported in the *British Medical Journal* and *The Lancet* within a month. Lawrie had referred to the commission appointed in 1888 by the Nizam's Government to make experiments on the effect of chloroform. This was to become known as the First Hyderabad Chloroform Commission, the members of which were Lawrie's own colleagues in Hyderabad.

"Surgeon-Major Lawrie, M.D., the Principal of the School, delivered a short address on the occasion, in the course of which he said the male and female students at that institution enjoyed, in many respects, practical advantages of which very few European schools could boast. They had made experiments with reference to the effects of chloroform, which had conclusively decided a question which has been in dispute ever since chloroform was first introduced. They had killed with chloroform 128 full-grown pariah dogs averaging over 20 lb. weight each. . . . This does not represent a tithe of the experiments they actually performed, which really amounted to several hundreds, as they varied the dose and the method of administering the chloroform in every possible way, and tested the value of artificial respiration in nearly every case by reviving the dogs over and over again after the breathing had stopped, and before the heart ceased beating. . . . The speaker added that, in the 40,000 or 50,000 administrations which he had superintended, he had never seen the heart injuriously or dangerously affected by chloroform. He had no doubt deaths would go on occurring until the London schools, which of course influence the whole world, either entirely changed their principles and ignored the heart in chloroform administration, or else confined themselves exclusively to the use of an anaesthetic like ether, which, with all its disadvantages, they know how to manage."[6,7]

Lawrie, with his reliance upon Simpson's and Syme's experience and methods, based his argument on very flimsy, dubious and unreliable grounds. It has been shown in another essay,[8] with plenty of supporting evidence, that Simpson's statistics were unreliable, if not actually dishonest. He described a death on the table in one of his own patients given chloroform, with the remark that it was the first such occurrence that he had seen in all his twenty-two years' experience of the agent. This was, quite definitely, not true. Syme, when he gave his dogmatic lecture about the safety of chloroform, had had a total experience of about two thousand cases;[9] his arguments were therefore untrustworthy. Chloroform has never been accused of, regularly, causing more than one death in every one or two thousand administrations. Moreover, Syme facilely assumed that, because at the time he spoke there had been thirteen deaths in London and only one in Edinburgh, chloroform administered in Scotland was thirteen times as safe as it was in England. Hence his condescending offer to teach the London doctors how to use it properly! He conveniently, and not very intelligently, ignored the fact that the population of London was, at the time, more than thirteen times as large as that of Edinburgh. Moreover, he had condensed the whole of his dissertation on anaesthesia into ten minutes — which is a fair indication of the extent of his knowledge of the subject.

Lawrie obviously did not know, or care to consider, these facts and he always looked upon Syme as infallible, and regarded his classical lecture as eternally and immutably true — a thing to which nothing could be added and from which nothing could be taken away. When Lawrie was using his own experience as a basis for his arguments he was on much more trustworthy ground, for his own anaesthetics far outnumbered those of Syme. We can discount very heavily the guesswork statistics of his initial speech: his own words "40,000 or 50,000 administrations" showed that he had no accurate idea of how many anaesthetics he had really given or supervised. It must have been a large number but, with a margin for error of some ten thousand cases it is clear that no careful records had been kept or consulted. Such an omission almost invariably would lead to a gross over-estimate of the numbers.

He did begin to keep careful notes of all the chloroform cases, and was able to give details of such cases at the Afzulgunj Hospital in Hyderabad.[10] The chloroform was administered for the whole of the month of April 1898 by a third year medical student at the Hyderabad Medical School. Normally this duty was entrusted to fourth year students but this had not been possible during the month since they were all out in the districts on "plague duty". In this one month 221 anaesthetics had been given, strictly according to Syme's method; 88 patients had received "chloroform analgesia" for minor operations. Lawrie was, therefore, accumulating considerable experience on which to base his views. He finished his article thus:

"We at Hyderabad have always said that if students in India can be taught to give chloroform with guaranteed safety, *a fortiori* the splendid men who study in the London medical schools with all their superior advantages can be taught to do the same."

Nothing if not controversial! However, it is to Lawrie's great credit that he did keep anaesthetic records eventually. He did this partly to teach his students but, mainly, because doubt had been cast upon his figures which, at first sight, seemed fantastic. Considering the above record of one month's work they were not so apocryphal as they then appeared.

Soon the first hint of opposition to Lawrie's teachings was published in *The Lancet*, referring to the remarks Lawrie had made at the Hyderabad prize-giving, and to the investigation that he had reported.

"Mr. Lawrie, as a disciple of Simpson and Syme, arrives at conclusions consonant with the teaching of those great clinicians, but utterly at variance with the experience alike of experiment and practice as carried out in Europe. We should require more than the scanty statements of experiments performed upon dogs. ... The primary syncope it is rarely, if ever, possible to induce in dogs, although, unfortunately, it is this form of heart failure which does occur in human beings, and which it is almost impossible to remedy. While welcoming the attention paid to the subject by the Hyderabad Chloroform Commission, we cannot but feel that, should the Commission inculcate a disregard of the heart as a factor in chloroform dangers, it will do harm and provoke a slipshod carelessness in the use of that valuable anaesthetic, which must in the long-run do damage to the cause the Commission has espoused."[11]

Now battle had been joined. *The Lancet*, quite rightly, wanted more detailed information. It had asked for the evidence, and not the verdict alone. Moreover, it wanted good evidence which could be assessed by everyone. The weakness of this, the First Hyderabad Choroform Commission, was that a doctrine which was contrary to all practical experience in Europe (and therefore, on the face of it, improbable) was suddenly put forward by a local body of somewhat obscure and unknown men. Their competence as impartial experimenters had yet to be established, and their leader was biased in favour of one answer — and no other — to the question under investigation. Certainly, they had transferred the results of their few animal experiments to human practice, and were dogmatic. In other words, there cropped up yet again the old fallacy of the effect of cantharides on the hedgehog.[12]

One of the difficulties in following the verbose and complicated byways of this controversy arises because of the slowness with which letters, at the time, travelled between India and England. By the time a reply had been received from Lawrie to one letter, other, related correspondence had accumulated in the journals.

Lawrie's reply to *The Lancet's* comments started with an excellent debating point, and he added a clever footnote which showed that, as a controversialist, he was of no mean calibre.

"... the writer states that 'all those who are familiar with chloroform are well aware that syncope, when primary, as a rule supervenes in the initial stages of inhalation, ...' and that unfortunately it is the primary form of chloroform heart failure which occurs in human beings, and which it is almost impossible to remedy."

Lawrie's footnote said:

"To be honest this sentence should run: 'All those who are familiar with *deaths from* chloroform *in human subjects*' — which I am not. — E.L."

His letter, then, continued.

"I have no wish to say anything to give offence to those who hold the same view as the writer of the annotation, but I hold that those views are wrong, and that there is no such thing as chloroform syncope.

"It is conceivable that syncope may occur in the initial stages of inhalation of chloroform, but in the course of a very large experience I have never met with a single instance of such an accident, and if it ever does occur it cannot be due to chloroform poisoning, though it might be caused by fright or shock.... On the other hand it is equally intelligible that syncope may be induced if an operation be commenced in the initial stages of chloroform administration, before the patient is rendered insensible to shock by being brought fully under its influence.... *The Lancet* asserts that the statements made in my address are utterly at variance with the experience alike of experiment and practice as carried out in Europe. They are, nevertheless, based on the principles taught by Syme and Simpson ... and long before the Hyderabad Commission was formed I had satisfied myself that they were entirely true....

"Our contention is that if the administration is ever pushed far enough to cause the heart to show signs of danger, the limits of safety have already been exceeded, and a fatal result must almost inevitably ensue. So far as disregarding the heart as a factor in chloroform dangers, we say that any affection of the heart, either direct or indirect, is the one danger to avoid. But we say, further, that the respiration invariably gives warnings when a dangerous point is approached, and consequently that it is possible to avert all risk to the heart by devoting the entire attention to the respiration during chloroform administration.

"... if *The Lancet* will not accept the conclusions of the Hyderabad Commission, it is incumbent on it to urge the appointment of a European or joint European and American Commission, composed of men of wide experience in chloroform, to confirm or disprove them."[13]

The Editor of *The Lancet* replied to this letter without delay.

"It is a matter of regret that, instead of complying with our request for fuller information, Mr. Lawrie has contented himself with mere dogmatic assertion and iteration of his former statements.... Mr. Lawrie has never seen a death from chloroform in the initial stages of narcosis; but he seems to forget that others, whose authority we are bound to accept, have done so ... Mr. Lawrie bases his conclusions upon premises the value of which we must decline to accept until full publicity be given to the last detail of the modes in which the Hyderabad Commission pursued its researches."[14]

The reply which *The Lancet* received from Lawrie some three months later (virtually "by return of post" when we remind ourselves of the distances, and slow transport, involved) was unequivocal, dramatic, and effective.

"I am directed by his Highness the Nizam's Government to offer *The Lancet*, as the leading medical journal, £1,000 to send out a representative to repeat the experiments of the Hyderabad Chloroform Commission, and make any others with the Commission that you may suggest.... The Nizam's Government has been advised that if the experiments are continued and amplified by the Hyderabad Commission, associated with a trained scientist, whose position and attainments will ensure the acceptance of his opinions by the profession, the subject might be threshed out thoroughly, and the question whether chloroform does or does not affect the heart directly, and other questions connected with it, might be settled once and for all. . . . The Hyderabad Commission undertake to place themselves entirely at his disposal and will act under his direction. The Commission will provide all instruments and appliances and everything which may be required for the experiments, and will, without bias, do all in their power to assist the representative of *The Lancet* in arriving at the truth."[15]

This reply, in effect, said "Very well. You will not accept our findings because we are obscure and unknown. So, let there be another Commission. Send out to India, as the Nizam's guest, any scientist with a world-wide reputation; the choice of this man is yours. He can repeat the previous work and extend it if he wishes. Everything he requires will be provided; the Nizam guarantees all the expenses." It was a princely offer; after all, £1,000 was a very large sum in those days.

The Lancet accepted the offer at once, and named the man chosen to be its representative. We might note however, that the Nizam's munificence was not to provide that which Lawrie had sought earlier, namely "a European or joint European and American Commission, composed of men of wide experience in chloroform".[13] Instead, one man (albeit an expert of international repute) was to be chosen to journey to Hyderabad (where the chloroformists were very much men of experience even if they did have decided views about the matter to be investigated) and, there, to carry out, and mainly repeat, the First Hyderabad Commission's experiments in, virtually, the same circumstances as before, amidst and with the assistance of the original Commissioners themselves. Further, the man the Editor chose had been a medical student contemporary with Lawrie at Edinburgh.[1] All things considered, and with the benefit of hindsight, we can see that this was not the best way to set up the ultimate in impartial investigations into the safe use of chloroform anaesthesia. The Nizam's money could, in truth, have been used in a more effective way. At the time, however, *The Lancet* saw no reason to cavil with the Nizam's offer which had been set out by Lawrie.

"This offer we have cheerfully accepted . . . in accordance with the Nizam's desire that we should select a man who is not only a trained scientist, but one whose position and attainments will ensure the acceptance of his opinions by the profession, we have requested Dr. Lauder Brunton, F.R.S., to act as our representative, and he has consented to set out for Hyderabad on Oct. 4th, which is the earliest possible opportunity.* Dr. Lauder Brunton has not only devoted much time to pharmacological work for more than twenty years, his first contribution on the action of nitrite of amyl having appeared in our columns of 1867; but the fact that his large work on 'Pharmacology and Therapeutics,' which appears also in an American edition, has been translated into French, and is now being translated into German, Italian and Spanish, shows that he is regarded as an authority in other countries as well as our own. It may perhaps be considered a farther advantage that in his work Dr. Lauder Brunton has very decidedly stated that one of the dangers resulting from chloroform is death by stoppage of the heart. 'Audi alteram partem'† is the motto of an important section of *The Lancet*; and we think that by getting both opinions regarding the effect of chloroform on the heart represented on the Commission, as they will be by Dr. Lauder Brunton and Surgeon-Major Lawrie, we are more likely to obtain a correct conclusion. The question whether chloroform paralyses the heart or not is one of the greatest possible practical importance, for upon its correct solution the lives of thousands of people and the happiness of thousands of families may depend. . . . It may not be possible to work out completely all the questions which may arise, but if the Hyderabad Commission, with the aid of Dr. Lauder Brunton, can settle definitely the question whether chloroform does or does not affect the heart directly, a most important practical object will have been obtained by means of the Nizam's generous offer."[16]

After this, there was an interval of nearly three months silence on the subject. Then came some astonishing, if not shattering news. *The Lancet* published, verbatim, a telegram which it had just received from Dr. Lauder Brunton in Hyderabad.

"Four hundred and ninety dogs, horses, monkeys, goats, cats and rabbits used. One hundred and twenty with manometer. All records photographed. Numerous observations on every individual animal. Results most instructive. Danger from chloroform is asphyxia or overdose; none whatever heart direct."[17]

The Lancet added, with a certain amount of pique,

"These results apparently indicate such a complete reversal of the view held by Dr. Lauder Brunton at the time he left England — that one of the dangers resulting from chloroform is death by stoppage of the heart — that the details of the experiments made by Dr. Brunton, and the reasons for the conclusions he has evidently arrived at, will be awaited with the greatest interest by the profession."

At first sight, it seemed that the First Hyderabad Commission's findings had been correct after all.

---

* This could not have been more than three weeks, or so after the receipt of Lawrie's letter by *The Lancet*, which must be some indication of Brunton's keenness to participate.

† This may be translated as "Hear both sides".

Dr. Thomas Lauder Brunton had left England on October 4th, 1889, and had arrived in Hyderabad on the 21st of the same month. The Second Hyderabad Commission, backed by his reputation and experience, began its work two days later, and for the following fifty-seven days until the 18th December, started work at seven o'clock in the morning and continued, each day, until five in the evening.[18] It had been originally supposed that Brunton would have been President of the Commission.

"When I arrived at Hyderabad, with characteristic generosity Lawrie wished to make me President of the Commission, but I felt that Lawrie's position in Hyderabad, the high esteem in which he was held by the Nizam and everyone in authority, as well as the fact that it was he who had originated the idea, clearly pointed Lawrie himself out as the proper man for President. In this Sir Gerald Bomford and all the other members of the Commission thoroughly concurred."[3]

Thus the Commission was headed by a decidedly biased person instead of, as *The Lancet* had surely hoped, their impartial and expert experimenter. Certainly *The Lancet* treated Brunton's telegram with a wise and cautious reserve.

"The limited space available in a telegraphic message prevented Dr. Lauder Brunton from giving any details of his experiments upon chloroform, and it is altogether premature to argue a question still *sub judice*. . . . It then becomes our duty to urge upon readers that the research which Dr. Lauder Brunton has undertaken is one not lightly dealt with . . . and it would be certainly wholly unjustifiable to relax any of the precautions and care at present adopted by practical anaesthetists as necessary when dealing with chloroform."[19]

The long hours which the Commission spent in the animal laboratory, in the stifling heat, carrying out a rapid succession of experiments on a variety of animals could hardly be thought of as being ideal conditions in which to perform such important research, the results of which were awaited eagerly by, virtually, the whole of the medical world. That the experiments were carried out in this way could well have been due to the impatience and driving force of the impetuous Lawrie: it can hardly be doubted that Lawrie's enthusiasm and his absolute conviction that his view was right must have had an unjudicial effect upon the famous physiologist. It really was both premature and ill-advised for Brunton to send his telegram to *The Lancet* so soon. I have no doubt that every word of his telegram was literally true, but it was, nonetheless, misleading. All that the Commission had shown was that sudden heart failure had not occurred in about 500 animals and this had nothing to do with its frequency in human

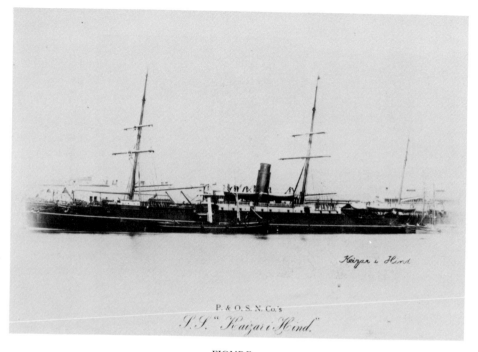

P. & O. S. N. Co.'s

S.S. "Kaizar i Hind."

FIGURE 71

Lauder Brunton travelled to India, by way of Brindisi in Italy, where he boarded this splendid P & O liner, the *Kaizar i Hind* (*Empress of India*) which, at the time, was one of the most luxurious of the "posh" liners. She was one of the first of the Company's liners to be fitted with air-conditioning.

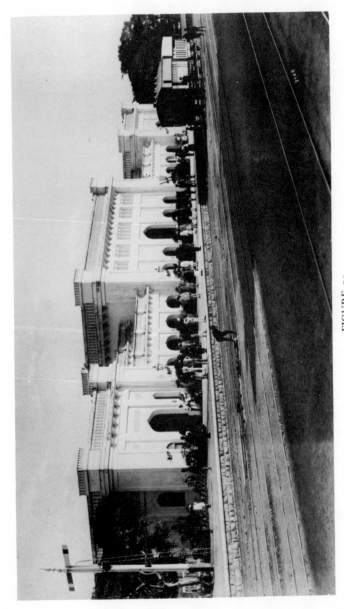

FIGURE 72

The railway station at Hyderabad where Brunton arrived from Bombay to start work for the Hyderabad Chloroform Commission on behalf of *The Lancet*. He soon found himself in very difficult circumstances indeed.

beings which, anyway, was not met with more frequently than one in two thousand cases or so.

Lawrie had, at least, allowed some fifteen years to elapse from the date of his first appointment as a resident hospital surgeon (by which time he had been more than convinced by Syme's teachings) until the time when he threw down the gauntlet to the world. Brunton, regrettably, could not even wait until the work of the Commission was finished and digested. His telegram was actually in print, in *The Lancet*, on the forty-sixth day of the Commission's laboratory investigations. Following soon after its cautious and reserved response to Brunton's telegram, *The Lancet* printed an account of a splendid dinner given in honour of the Commission by the local Governor, or Nawab.[20] Banquets such as this, and the princely receptions and entertainment offered to Lauder Brunton, might well have been among the factors which tended to obscure his judgement.

The Report of the Second Hyderabad Chloroform Commission was published in two forms. Beginning in January 1890, *The Lancet* printed the report in five, more or less monthly instalments.[18, 21, 22, 23, 24] A year or so later, the Report was published as a single volume.[25] That the two versions of the Report are not identical can, largely, be explained on the grounds of *The Lancet's* editorial decisions about which material was considered to be of greatest practical importance. However, some of the discrepancies between *The Lancet's* instalments and the single-volume Report which appeared after more than a year's delay require a different explanation, of which more later.

The first instalment was preceded by an editorial in *The Lancet* which reflected the journal's unease about the Commission's findings.

"The practical outcome of the research would appear to be that deaths from chloroform are not inevitable. They are therefore preventable, and by due care in its administration they may be with certainty avoided. The conclusions of the Commission are sweeping, and without abundant evidence cannot be accepted."[26]

The Report itself, as published in *The Lancet*, first outlined the work of the earlier Hyderabad Chloroform Commission and the disappointing response with which its findings were greeted in most quarters; it then went on to explain how the Second Commission had come into existence. The members of the Second Commission were Surgeon Major Lawrie (as President) Dr. Lauder Brunton, Surgeon Major Gerald Bomford (of the Indian Medical Service, and who had been nominated to the Commission by the Government of India at the request of the Nizam's Government) and Dr. Rustomji (of the Nizam's Medical Service, and later referred to as Dr.

Rustomji D. Hakim). A Dr. Bomford acted as Secretary. These gentlemen were assisted by the members of the earlier Commission, namely Surgeon P. Hehir, Mr. J. A. Kelly and Dr. Arthur Chamarette. Dr. Gay also volunteered to help. Laconically, the account continued:

"The Commission is very much indebted to all the gentlemen mentioned, as well as to Mr. William Mayberry, who gave chloroform; . . ."

(Since the Nizam provided everything for the Commission it may be assumed that the hard-working Mr. Mayberry did not actually donate the chloroform, but must have administered it for the experiments instead.) The Commission began its work on the 23rd October, 1889 and worked daily from 7 a.m. until 5 p.m. every day except for Sundays and holidays. Within this time 430 animals were chloroformed in various circumstances, and their modes of death observed. The Nizam, himself, witnessed several of the experiments.

The Commission organised itself with military efficiency, into "The Committee" (which consisted of Brunton, Bomford, Hehir and Chamarette) and "The Subcommittee" (made up of Dr. Rustomji, Mr. Kelly and Dr. Gay, who were assisted by a number of medical students).

The "Committee" first performed 27 experiments designed to test the validity of the work of the First Commission and, this done, the Second Commission began its further work in earnest. The "Committee" conducted those experiments which required blood pressure recording apparatus, and

"The ordinary experiments, performed without recording apparatus, were then made over to the Subcommittee, which continued to work in the same room under the supervision of the Commission. . . . The experiments of the Subcommittee, together with the first twenty-eight performed by the Committee, form a total of 430 . . . 268 dogs and 31 monkeys were killed outright, and 86 dogs and 39 monkeys were subjected to artificial respiration at varying intervals after the natural respiration had been arrested with chloroform. The animals which were killed had chloroform administered to them in every possible way and under every conceivable condition. A large number of dogs were killed just as they were caught in the bazaars; others at various intervals after having heavy meals of meat or farinaceous food or fat; others fasting; others after the administration of Liebig's extract of meat, coffee, rectified spirits of wine or ammonia. Most of these animals were healthy, but some of them had cardiac disease, and in many the heart and other organs were rendered fatty by the previous administration of phosphorus. In a large number of cases morphine, strychnine, and atropine, singly and in combination were given by subcutaneous injection at intervals before the inhalation was begun. Chloroform was given with and without inhalers; in the vertical and recumbent positions; in glass and wooden boxes; in large and small doses; by being

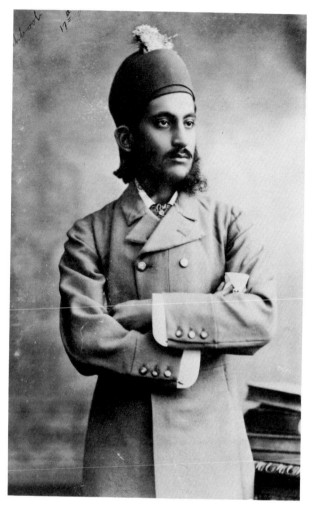

FIGURE 73

The Nizam of Hyderabad in 1890.

pumped into the trachea with bellows; and, in fact, in every way that could suggest itself to the Commission.

"The results in one respect are uniform. In every case where chloroform was pushed the respiration stopped before the heart. . . .

"The movement of the heart was in the first 66 cases of the Subcommittee tested by auscultation, but afterwards by a needle inserted through the chest wall into the organ, and the thoracic cavity was laid open when doubt existed."

The Committee performed 157 experiments with blood pressure recording apparatus, and said that almost every experiment included

"a variety of procedures which suggested themselves at the time as likely to elucidate something in the action of the different anaesthetics employed.

"In a certain number of cases the animal died accidentally before it was ready to be attached to the manometer. . . . The majority of the experiments were made upon dogs or monkeys, and a few upon horses, goats, cats and rabbits.

"The experiments of the Committee were designed to show the effect upon the blood pressure, heart and respiration of the inhalation of chloroform, ether, and the A.C.E. mixture administered in various ways and under varying conditions. . . .

"Complete stoppage of respiration always means that an over-dose has been administered, and the over-dose may have been so great as to produce a very prolonged after-fall of blood pressure, and may thus render restoration impossible. . . .

"The time which may be allowed to pass with impunity before commencing artificial respiration also seems to vary considerably. . . .

"In order to test the alleged danger from shock during chloroform administration, the Committee peformed a very large number of those operations which are reputed to be particularly dangerous in this connexion — such as extraction of teeth, evulsion of nails, section of the muscles of the eye, snipping of the skin of the anus, &c . . . but in no case in any stage of anaesthesia was there anything even suggestive of syncope or failure of the heart's action.

"The conclusion, then, is this: Chloroform has no power of increasing the tendency to either shock or syncope during operations. If shock or syncope from any cause does occur, it prevents, rather than aggravates, the dangers of chloroform inhalation. . . .

"The failure of the heart, if such it can be called, instead of being a danger to the animal, proved to be a positive safeguard, by preventing the absorption of the residual chloroform and its distribution throughout the system. . . .

"It corresponds to those cases, which are so often reported, in which dangerous failure of the heart is said to have occurred some minutes after the administration of the chloroform has been discontinued, and which are sometimes restored, and sometimes not, by artificial respiration. There is nothing at all sudden about the failure of the heart in these cases, but the attention of the chloroformist, which has been wandering, is suddenly called to the fact that the patient is apparently dead."

I have edited this part of the report quite drastically, but do not believe that I have, in so doing, altered the message the Commission wished, in 1890, to convey.

The section of the Report entitled "Accidental Deaths" put forward the Commission's views on how these happened during their experiments.

"The fatal result was brought about either by neglecting to watch the condition of the respiration during or after the administration of chloroform, especially while the carotid artery was being exposed, or from a reckless administration of chloroform in the endeavour to check or prevent struggles. In all the cases of accidental death the usual chloroformist was absent, and no one was attending to the chloroform. The notes would have been more complete if someone could have watched the condition of the animal and noted the gradual but unheeded cessation of respiration without calling attention to it. As it is, one has to be content with the remark that the breathing was noticed to have stopped at some particular time, but there is nothing to throw any light upon the condition during the important period that immediately preceded this discovery. A similar hiatus appears in the account of accidental deaths in the human subject and is unavoidable. These cases are probably identical with those instances referred to by Snow, 'in which animals died in a sudden and what was thought unaccountable manner whilst chloroform was given to prevent the pain and struggles which would be occasioned by physiological experiments'. The death was not really sudden, but only rapid, and the result of reckless administration of concentrated vapour in the first instance, and careless neglect of the condition of the respiration in the second. There is no evidence whatever that a single one of them was due to paralysis or sudden stoppage of the heart, as Snow assumes to have been the case."

The Lancet's first instalment of the Commission's Report ended with a section entitled "Practical Conclusions", a list of 14 points which "may fairly be deduced from the experiments recorded in this report".

"I. The recumbent position on the back and absolute freedom of respiration are essential.

"II. If during an operation the recumbent position on the back cannot, from any cause, be maintained during chloroform administration, the utmost attention to the respiration is necessary to prevent asphyxia or an overdose. If there is any doubt whatever about the state of respiration, the patient should be at once restored to the recumbent position on the back.

"III. To ensure absolute freedom of respiration, tight clothing of every kind, either on the neck, chest, or abdomen, is to be strictly avoided; and no assistants or bystanders should be allowed to exert pressure on any part of the patient's thorax or abdomen, even though the patient be struggling violently. If struggling does occur, it is always possible to hold the patient down by pressure on the shoulders,

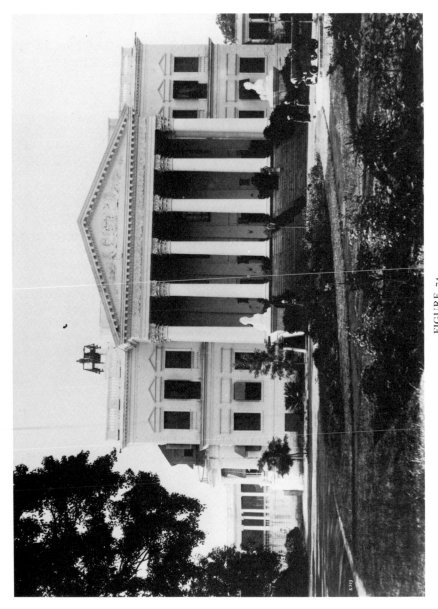

FIGURE 74

The Residency in Hyderabad. In this building (the residence of the British Ambassador) was the hospital in which much of Lawrie's work was done.

pelvis, or legs without doing anything which can by any possibility interfere with the free movements of respiration.

"IV. An apparatus is not essential, and ought not to be used, as, being made to fit the face, it must tend to produce asphyxia. Moreover, it is apt to take up part of the attention which is required elsewhere. In short, no matter how it is made, it introduces an element of danger into the administration. A convenient form of inhaler is an open cone or cap with a little absorbent cotton inside at the apex.

"V. At the commencement of inhalation care should be taken, by not holding' the cap too close over the mouth and nose, to avoid exciting, struggling, or holding the breath. If struggling or holding the breath do occur, great care is necessary to avoid an over-dose during the deep inspirations which follow. When quiet breathing is ensured as the patient begins to go over, there is no reason why the inhaler should not be applied close to the face; and all that is then necessary is to watch the cornea and to see that the respiration is not interfered with.

"VI. In children, crying ensures free admission of chloroform into the lungs; but as struggling and holding the breath can hardly be avoided, and one or two whiffs of chloroform may be sufficient to produce complete insensibility, they should always be allowed to inhale a little fresh air during the first deep inspirations which follow. In any struggling persons, but especially in children, it is essential to remove the inhaler after the first or second deep inspiration, as enough chloroform may have been inhaled to produce deep anaesthesia, and this may only appear, or may deepen, after the chloroform is stopped. Struggling is best avoided in adults by making them blow out hard after each inspiration during the inhalation.

"VII. The patient is, as a rule, anaesthetised and ready for the operation to be commenced when unconscious winking is no longer produced by touching the surface of the eye with the tip of the finger. The anaesthetic should never under any circumstances be pushed until respiration stops; but when once the cornea is insensitive, the patient should be kept gently under by occasional inhalations, and not be allowed to come out and renew the stage of struggling and resistance.

"VIII. As a rule, no operation should be commenced until the patient is fully under the influence of the anaesthetic, so as to avoid all chance of death from surgical shock or fright.

"IX. The administrator should be guided as to the effect entirely by the respiration. His only object, while producing anaesthesia, is to see that the respiration is not interfered with.

"X. If possible, the patient's chest and abdomen should be exposed during chloroform inhalation so that the respiratory movements can be seen by the administrator. If anything interferes with the respiration in any way, however slightly, even if this occurs at the very commencement of the administration, if the breath is held, or if there is stertor, the inhalation should be stopped until the breathing is natural again. This may sometimes create delay and inconvenience with inexperienced administrators, but experience will make any administrator so familiar with the respiratory functions under chloroform that he will in a short time know almost by intuition whether anything is going wrong, and be able to put it right without delay before any danger arises.

"XI. If the breathing becomes embarrassed, the lower jaw should be pulled, or pushed from behind the angles, forward, so that the lower teeth protrude in front of the upper. This raises the epiglottis and frees the larynx. At the same time it is well to assist the respiration artificially until the embarrassment passes off.

"XII. If by any accident the respiration stops, artificial respiration should be commenced at once, while an assistant lowers the head and draws forward the tongue with catch-forceps, by Howard's method, assisted by compression and relaxation of the thoracic walls. Artificial respiration should be continued until there is no doubt whatever that natural respiration is completely re-established.

"XIII. A small dose of morphia may be injected sub-cutaneously before chloroform inhalation, as it helps to keep the patient in a state of anaesthesia in prolonged operations. There is nothing to show that atropine does any good in connexion with the administration of chloroform, and it may do a very great deal of harm.

"XIV. Alcohol may be given with advantage before operations under chloroform, provided it does not cause excitement, and merely has the effect of giving a patient confidence and steadying the circulation."

These conclusions are all sound enough. Very few anaesthetists would have disapproved of them if they were thought of as simple instructions for giving chloroform. None of the conclusions, however, appear to have any marked connection with the weeks of patient laboratory work undertaken by the Commission.

Lauder Brunton appears to have been infected by the prevailing atmosphere of enthusiasm and optimism to such an extent that he completely overlooked his position as an impartial referee and assessor. His misleading — albeit true — telegram sent off to *The Lancet* even before the experiments were finished is a good example of this fervour. In addition, Brunton appended his name to the Report which in its conclusions dropped all mention of his laborious, experimental work on animals, and merely became an elementary lecture on chloroform administration in human beings. Now Brunton, for all his experience as a physician and physiologist, had probably given few, if any, anaesthetics to humans since he had been a student in the early eighteen-sixties.

The speed at which the Report was compiled and published in instalment form is relevant. The experimental work of the Commission continued until December 18th, and the first instalment (which was the most important one) was printed in *The Lancet* a month later. Brunton's outward journey from London to Hyderabad took seventeen days or so, and, presumably, the Report took about this length of time to make the return journey. This means that the substance of the Report was written within a fortnight. (I suppose that it may, in essence, have been written before the Commission actually completed its work; under the circumstances its conclusions must have been quite predictable to those involved at the outset.) Brunton, himself, said that "The amount of experimental work we did in three months was so great it would really have taken a man his whole time for three years to work out all that was shown by the tracings".[1] This was written 26 years later and was not very exact; the sharp edges of memory had become blunted by the passage of time for the laboratory work did not actually take 3 months, but rather less than two. The three years needed to work out all the tracings was also, no doubt, too generous an estimate. Still, there was evidently a very great deal to be done — and the Report was written in just two weeks!

Here again we see the impetuosity of Lawrie, who could not wait. Brunton's work, and the Nizam's generosity in paying for the Commission were pushed aside and, to a large extent, wasted. What emerged was just a re-hash of Syme's casual lecture on chloroform and how it should be administered. It is significant that the last of the practical conclusions, as published in *The Lancet*, ends with words very similar to those which Syme used thirty years earlier.[27]

"... chloroform may be given in any case requiring an operation with perfect ease and absolute safety so as to do good without the risk of evil."

Truly, *The Lancet* hit the nail right on the head when it stated, on its publication of the Report

"The Commission owed its existence to Surgeon Major Lawrie's veneration for his late teacher, Professor Syme, and his desire to prove the correctness of Syme's teaching ..."[26]

As mentioned earlier, the Report which was published in *The Lancet* differed from that which appeared a year or more later, in 1891, in book form.[25] This was published at the Nizam's expense by the Times of India Steam Press, and was distributed to major medical libraries throughout the world.

The book form contained two sections which were, virtually, unpublished by *The Lancet*, and that journal published one section not included in the book. *The Lancet* omitted much of the detailed, longhand description of each of the Committee's experiments with blood pressure recording apparatus (which appeared in the book) but included a lengthy section of

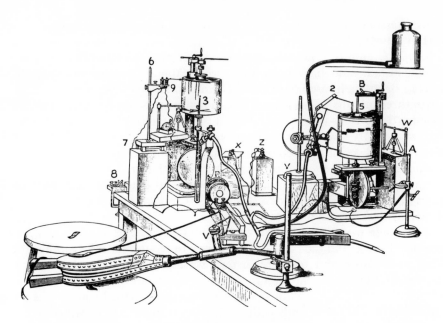

FIGURE 75

This must be one of the most complicated diagrams ever drawn to simplify the description of an experiment. It shows the manometer, and other, apparatus employed by the members of the Committee of the Second Hyderabad Chloroform Commission during their investigations of the effects of chloroform on the heart and respiration of dogs, and other animals. The description in *The Lancet* was as follows:

"The apparatus stands on a solid teak table. In front is seen a strong upright for supporting a Bernard's dog holder. Close behind the upright is a wooden burette-holder, bent almost to a horizontal position. This was used to support the elongated glass bulb connected with the arterial cannula, and to prevent any drag being exerted upon it. Y is almost hidden by the upright, and is supported by a long needle above the Y-tube, which it indicates. From the Y-tube go two white tubes to the two manometers; 2 indicates Fick's manometer; 3 is fastened above the mercurial manometer, against the tracing on Ludwig's kymograph, above the clockwork of which 9 is fastened; 6 indicates the magnetic time-marker, and is raised on a large block of wood to a proper height; on a small block of wood at the bottom of the instrument is seen the watch of the observer; 7 is the Dubois-Reymond key, by which the time-marker is worked; R is a Dubois-Reymond's coil for irritating nerves; 8, the key by which contact is made and broken; X is a Leclanche battery for the time-marker, and Z is a bichromate cell for the coil; 5 indicates the tracing on Fick's kymograph, and W the clockwork of the instrument; A and B are two of Marey's tambours connected together. The lever of A was connected occasionally by a thread with a needle fixed in the heart or diaphragm of the animal, and the movement being transmitted to A was recorded by it on the cylinder of Fick's kymograph. V indicates the valve used with the bellows for artificial respiration. It is fixed to the nozzle of the bellows by a kind of splint made of wood and cork. Across the top of the photograph and down its centre extends the indiarubber tube conveying soda solution to the apparatus from the vessel fixed against the wall." (*Lancet* (1890), **1**, 1386) more or less representative tracings obtained by the Committee (which did not appear in the book).

The book version contained one section which *The Lancet* could not have published. This section began with the text of Syme's original lecture given in 1885[27] and this was followed by numerous articles — reprinted word for word — which had a bearing on the Commission's work, and which had been published in the interval between the appearance of *The Lancet's* first instalment, in 1889, and the production of the report in book form by the Times of India Steam Press. Some of the articles included in this section were critical of the Commission; others supported it. Lawrie, almost certainly, must have edited this section of the book himself, and Brunton, who had returned to London, would have had little or no part in deciding which articles were included, and which were not.

The most important extras to be found in the book version of the Report are at the very end of the volume, following the last of the fourteen "Practical Conclusions" which had first appeared in *The Lancet* more than a year earlier.

"The practical conclusions are reproduced here in their original form. They were written before the Commission had time to realise the full meaning of their experimental data, or opportunity to put them to the test of clinical experience. They were not regarded as final by the Commission as it was hoped and expected that surgeons and physiologists would examine the tracings and descriptions of the experiments for themselves, and draw their own conclusions from them."

This does not accord with the professed purpose of the Commission which Lawrie, himself, had referred to when he announced the Nizam's offer of support.

"the Nizam's Government has been advised that if the experiments are continued and amplified by the Hyderabad Commission, associated with a trained scientist, . . . the subject might be threshed out thoroughly, and the question whether chloroform does or does not affect the heart directly, and other questions connected with it, might be settled once for all."[15]

The book form of the Report then compared the main points of Syme's original suggestions with the conclusions that the Commission had reached as a result of its work. We must not be surprised to learn that the Commission was completely in unison with Syme!

The final passage of the book version reads as follows:

"The report thus ends by showing how thoroughly the Hyderabad Commission has succeeded in proving that the late Professor Syme's principles of chloroform administration are right. This is the most fitting tribute the Commission can pay to the genius and wisdom of the illustrious surgeon, who, by his teaching and example, elevated and ennobled British surgery and paved the way for the new era inaugurated while yet he had full time to appreciate it, by his equally illustrious son-in-law Sir Joseph Lister."

By the time the Report was published in this form Brunton must have had some misgivings about the validity of the Commission's views. Nonetheless, his name was still appended to the later version of the Report (which, incidentally, included details of one experiment — number 186 in the series — performed in Hyderabad on March 6th, 1890 which was several months after Brunton had returned to the United Kingdom).

There are several reasons which, with the benefit of hindsight, may have led to Lauder Brunton's finding himself in an unenviable, if not impossible position during his time in Hyderabad. Indeed, it is unlikely that any one person could have achieved the objectives which *The Lancet's* Editors must have had in mind when, recalling his earlier, contrary views to those of Syme, they nominated him as "not only a trained scientist, but one whose position and attainments will ensure the acceptance of his opinions by the profession."[16] Brunton, I am sure, recognised vanity for the impostor it was and is, but he would hardly have been human if he did not derive some pleasure and pride from being described to the world at large in such glowing terms.

Against Brunton's obvious qualification for the task he was set, one must put several factors. It was a pity that Brunton had been a contemporary medical student with Lawrie at Edinburgh, and that he obviously had pleasant memories of the times they spent together.[3] This may have inhibited Brunton from challenging or denying the views which Lawrie held on chloroform with all the fervour of a zealot. There can be no real doubt that Lawrie, personally, intended the Second Commission to confirm the results of Syme's teaching and, thus, the results of the First Commission's work. This was, to him, exactly the same as "proving the question once and for all". Lawrie would have found himself in a most embarrassing position if the Commission did not confirm Syme's teaching which he had proclaimed so loudly for so long. He, also, would have been in an invidious position *vis à vis* the Nizam if the results of the First Commission had been shown to be incorrect. Lawrie enjoyed the Nizam's complete confidence, and had persuaded him to pay for the First Commission's work.

It is a pity that Brunton did not accept the offer of being the Commission's President, and that he insisted on Lawrie as President instead. The authority which Brunton might have gained in the eyes of his co-workers could have been most useful. Lawrie, as President, was allowed to direct the investigations more or less as he pleased. The Commission started its task only two days after Brunton had arrived in Hyderabad, which did not allow much time for him to acclimatise or familiarise himself with the conditions in which he was to work. There was also insufficient time to prepare a well-thought-out protocol for the investigations, and it is hardly surprising to read in the Report that things were done often on the spur of the moment if they were thought to have a bearing on chloroform's action on the heart, and that the methods used were changed from time to time.

The virtual repetition of the First Commission's work in the presence of the Commissioners who had themselves done that work could be considered to be a subtle exercise in brainwashing inflicted on Brunton surrounded, as he was, by a majority of people who were under Lawrie's influence and who had far, far greater practical experience with chloroform than Brunton. It is surprising that nine or so accidental deaths were allowed to occur during experiments which were designed to show the complete safety of chloroform. These were ascribed to carelessness or inattention by the administrator of the anaesthetics, but — and it is a big but — if nobody was attending to the animals' anaesthetics how did they know that the deaths were due to a respiratory cause and not of cardiac origin? Brunton, with all his training, must have considered this very elementary point but, presumably, was convinced by the facile explanations of his fellow Commissioners. It may well be that the investigators did experience deaths from primary cardiac failure during chloroform anaesthesia but failed, or were not prepared, to recognise it for what it really was.

Nonetheless, the perspective of history reveals that there were no villains in the story of the Second Hyderabad Chloroform Commission. Each and every one concerned was motivated by his own, personal interpretation of the facts available, and by the very highest ideals. But Brunton was "over a barrel".

REFERENCES

[1] Obituary (1915) *British Medical Journal*, **2**, 350–351.

[2] Obituary (1915) *Lancet*, **2**, 581.

[3] Brunton, L. (1915) The late Lieutenant-Colonel Edward Lawrie. *Lancet*, **2**, 624.

[4] Buxton, D. W. (1915) The late Lieutenant-Colonel Edward Lawrie, I.M.S. *Lancet*, **2**, 676.

[5] Annotation (1915) *Lancet*, **2**, 712.

[6] Annotation (1889) Hyderabad Medical School: Chloroform Inhalation. *Lancet*, **1**, 394.

[7] Annotation (1889) Chloroform administration. *British Medical Journal*, **1**, 429.

8 Sykes, W. S. (1960) *Essays on the First Hundred Years of Anaesthesia. Volume I.* London: Livingstone.
9 Sykes, W. S. (1960) *Essays on the First Hundred Years of Anaesthesia. Volume I.* London: Livingstone.
10 Lawrie, E. (1898) The production of chloroform anaesthesia. *Lancet*, **1**, 1681–1682.
11 Annotation (1889) The Hyderabad Commission on chloroform. *Lancet*, **1**, 438.
12 Sykes, W. S. (1960) *Essays on the First Hundred Years of Anaesthesia. Volume I.* London: Livingstone.
13 Lawrie, E. (1889) The Hyderabad Chloroform Commission. *Lancet*, **1**, 952–953.
14 Annotation (1889) Surgeon-Major Lawrie on the Hyderabad Commission. *Lancet*, **1**, 949.
15 Lawrie, E. (1889) The Hyderabad Chloroform Commission. *Lancet*, **2**, 601.
16 Annotation (1889) *The Lancet* and the Hyderabad Chloroform Commission. *Lancet*, **2**, 606.
17 Annotation (1889) *The Lancet* and the Hyderabad Chloroform Commission. *Lancet*, **2**, 1183.
18 Lawrie, E. (1890) Report of the Second Hyderabad Chloroform Commission. *Lancet*, **1**, 149–159.
19 Annotation (1889) The Hyderabad Chloroform Commission. *Lancet*, **2**, 1245.
20 Anonymous (1889) *The Lancet* and the Hyderabad Chloroform Commission. *Lancet*, **2**, 1245–1246.
21 Lawrie, E., Brunton, T. L., Bomford, G., & Hakim, R. D. (1890) The Hyderabad Chloroform Commissions. *Lancet*, **1**, 421–429.
22 Lawrie, E., Brunton, T. L., Bomford, G., & Hakim, R. D. (1890) The Hyderabad Chloroform Commissions. Report of the Second Commission. *Lancet*, **1**, 486–510.
23 Lawrie, E., Brunton, T. L., Bomford, G., & Hakim, R. D. (1890) The Hyderabad Chloroform Commission. The Report of the Second Commission. *Lancet*, **1**, 1140–1142.
24 Lawrie, E., Brunton, T. L., Bomford, G., & Hakim, R. D. (1890) The Report of the Second Hyderabad Chloroform Commission. *Lancet*, **1**, 1369–1388.
25 Lawrie, E., Brunton, T. L., Bomford, G., & Hakim, R. D. (1891) *Report of the Hyderabad Chloroform Commission.* Bombay: The Times of India Steam Press.
26 Editorial (1890) *Lancet*, **1**, 139.
27 Syme, J. (1855) Lectures on Clinical Surgery delivered during the winter session of 1854–55. *Lancet*, **1**, 55–57.

CHAPTER 18

IN SUPPORT OF LAWRIE AND HIS VIEWS

With the best will in the world, and after a most exhaustive search, I could only find one real argument in favour of Lawrie's teachings. That is his own, huge experience of the subject. We know, from his book,[1] that he had only one death in 17,300 cases during eight, almost nine, years, to which must be added an unknown, but undoubtedly large number (of cases, not deaths) anaesthetised with chloroform during the previous twenty years. This record is absolutely amazing, and almost unbelievably good. There is, however, no valid reason to doubt it.

This, then, is the *prima facie* evidence which seems to be almost impregnable and unanswerable. No wonder that Edward Lawrie was convinced that he knew all the answers. There must have been some very good reasons why Lawrie seemed to be so successful with his use of chloroform

A large number of people gave chloroform to a huge number of patients by all sorts of methods without ever encountering a death. Syme, for example, ran up a total of between five and six thousand such cases during his lifetime — Lawrie never tired of quoting this fact in support of the perfection of Syme's method. But one person whose experience Lawrie did not care to quote was Dr. Joseph Clover, the professional anaesthetist. He said, in 1871:

"I have administered chloroform more than seven thousand times, and ether, tetrachloride of carbon, ethylidenchlorid, the compound 'bichloride of methylene', and nitrous oxide, in four thousand other cases. I have never drawn out the tongue, and never lost a patient from any anaesthetic. . . . It is my habit when giving anaesthetics to watch the pulse as well as the breathing, and I am, therefore, better able to speak of the effect of chloroform upon the heart than those who disregard the pulse."[2]

Here, then, is the experience of a person who had conducted many more successful cases than Syme — and, what is more, had used the very method which Syme and Lawrie condemned as unsafe. Moreover, sixteen months later, when Clover's total must have increased considerably, his record was still free from deaths.

The average death rate, in Europeans, from sudden cardiac failure (that is the unpreventable deaths as opposed to the avoidable ones due to overdosage) was variously calculated as one in two thousand or so. Thus it would have been quite possible to have reached large numbers without encountering a death merely by good luck alone. I find no difficulty in believing such figures in the neighbourhood of five thousand: Syme's figures were of this order, and no one could call his happy-go-lucky method skilful. Clover, on the other hand, did have skill at his disposal — probably far much more than Lawrie, for he was not such a jack of all trades.

Lawrie's figures were, however, in a completely different class. They were so huge that it is quite impossible that mere good luck could have held out for so long. His first anaesthetic death occurred some twenty-seven years after he arrived in India and, during a large part of this time, he had administered or supervised chloroform anaesthesia for upwards of 2,000 operations each year. During a comprehensive search I found records of only five deaths under chloroform in India during the whole quarter of a century. It is not reasonable to suppose that news of all Indian deaths would have reached the British journals, but the interest in and the virulence of the controversy would have ensured that a good many of them did.

Clearly factors other than luck must have come into play.

The first of these which we might consider is the effect of racial difference. Was there anything in the mental or physical make-up of Eastern races which differed in some significant way from that of Europeans? Lawrie, himself, thought not. He wrote that he had given chloroform for seven years in the United Kingdom and for 22 years in India and had never noticed the slightest difference in susceptibility.[3] Since he qualified in 1867 and went to India five years later it is difficult to understand how he could have accumulated seven years' anaesthetic experience during this time, unless he counted two of his years as a senior student. He must have done this, but his opinion on such a point formed during his student years must have been of little objective value. In any event his opinion, like nearly all of his arguments, referred only to questions of chloroform overdosage.

(I am inclined to think that he was correct in this respect, physically at any rate. I never noticed any physical differences in the response to anaesthesia in different races, and I had a large experience of this in prisoner of war camp hospitals in Germany during World War Two. I gave anaesthetics to patients of forty-eight different nationalities and did not notice any racial peculiarities in the particular circumstances in which I found myself.)

Mental considerations are, probably, far more important in explaining why Lawrie (and other anaesthetists in India) had so very few fatalities under chloroform. Large among these factors was the fatalistic attitude of his Indian patients. Dr. J. F. W. Silk, of Guy's and King's College Hospitals in London, remarked:

"... it is, I believe, well known among Indian surgeons that the natives take chloroform remarkably well and that deaths, though not absolutely unknown, are very rare. For instance, Dr. Crawford, of the Madras General Hospital, says that the difference in mortality between India and Europe is not due to superiority of method, but to absence of fear and vast difference in temperament. Habit, custom and climate all tend to lessen the native's fear of losing consciousness."[4]

It may be difficult to appreciate what Dr. Silk meant by "habit" until one refers to the original statement. What Dr. Crawford (who used Syme's method for anaesthesia) actually had said was:

"... if once [they] are persuaded to enter a hospital they place themselves absolutely in the hands of the surgeon and feel no alarm or uneasiness either about the issue of the anaesthesia or the operation. Habit, custom, and climate all tend to lessen the native's fear of losing consciousness. He habitually takes opium and sees others go under its influence, and as he never hears of any deaths occurring under chloroform he has no reason to dread it."[5]

Arthur Neve, an Edinburgh-trained missionary surgeon in Kashmir, said that between 1882 and 1890 upwards of 11,000 operations had been performed at his hospital and he, himself, had witnessed the chloroform being administered in more than 3,000 of these.

"As far as the inhabitants of Central Asia and North India are concerned, chloroform may be regarded as a perfect anaesthetic. True, the beer drinking Tibetans occasionally struggle before succumbing to its influence, but of other races — Yarkandis, Hillmen, Pathans, Dards, Kasmiris, etc. — it may be said that to 99 per cent. chloroform may be given deeply and its administration prolonged without a drawback — no cardiac weakness, no bronchial irritation, very rarely signs of an overdose."[6]

That these psychological factors were real was borne out by the opinion of John Smyth, of the Madras General Hospital, who visited hospitals in the United Kingdom for the first time in twelve years.

"What struck me chiefly was the look of terror on the faces of most of the patients as they prepared to submit themselves to the anaesthetic — nothing could be in greater contrast with all this than the happy anticipation of freedom from pain which, I may say, characterises our patients in the East."[7]

Most of Lawrie's patients were Hindus or Mohammedans. Both of these groups had the ingrained fatalism of the East, in addition to the reverence which existed at that time for the white man, his knowledge and wisdom.

This would increase their confidence and lessen their fear. A large proportion of them were illiterate, so they could not read any reports of chloroform deaths! The Mohammedans were even more conditioned to fatalism by his religion — to them, if not to the Hindu, it was an article of faith. These factors, impalpable and invisible as they were, served as the very best preventives of primary cardiac failure; this is, no doubt, the reason why Lawrie all but never met with the condition in his whole, vast experience.

In addition to the psychological factors, the physical circumstances in India must also have played a part in ensuring Lawrie's success, although not everyone agreed at the time. An Indian chloroformist wrote, in 1894, "There is nothing in the 'clime' of Hyderabad which is favourable to the administration of chloroform . . . it is quite as easy to kill with chloroform here as it is in London or Philadelphia".[8] Leonard Hill, of The London Hospital, wrote:

"Surgeon-Lieutenant-Colonel Lawrie would have us believe that such a thing as chloroform syncope does not exist, and that European anaesthetists have to chronicle deaths from chloroform which roughly average 1 in 2,000 (many are never recorded), because in Europe the method is controlled by false teaching, and is inferior to that in India. Now the plain matter of fact is this. It is in India practically impossible to anaesthetise a dog with ether owing to the climate and rapidity of evaporation. It is the climate which likewise acts as a safeguard in chloroform anaesthesia, and prevents syncope."[9]

Hill exaggerated his argument, because ether can be used in hot climates, but there is truth in it nevertheless. Both ether and chloroform would have evaporated more quickly, which explains why Lawrie's heroic, drachm doses slopped on to the cone or mask at intervals did not have disastrous results. Heavy vapours would not linger around the patient's face as in the closed operating theatres of temperate climates — the Hyderabad theatre was open on three sides.

Another anaesthetist in India commented:

"I am convinced that our pure freely circulating air (for all operations are practically done in the open air); the dilute form in which the chloroform is necessarily administered owing to the high temperatures of the atmosphere; the constitutional peculiarities of our patients, the result of difference in food, clothing, and temperate habits — I say I am convinced that these different conditions have a great deal more to do in rendering chloroform anaesthesia safe here than any particular difference in the methods we adopt."[10]

There were, indeed, marked differences in diet between people in India and Europe. In India the intake of protein, especially of animal protein, was small — for economic and religious reasons. As late as 1944, Dr. K. E. Madan, of Lahore, wrote:

"While fully aware of the dangers of chloroform and the undesirability of its use, certain factors make chloroform less toxic and relatively safer in a healthy Indian than in a European. This is due to the Indian diet, which is principally carbohydrate and starch, in contrast to the predominantly nitrogenous diet of the West. The population in India is mainly vegetarian. . . . Under these dietetic conditions the livers of Indians are well replenished with glycogen. . . . From my long experience I am convinced that in strong, healthy, and active Indians living on rich carbohydrate diet the careful use of chloroform merely for inducing anaesthesia produces scarcely any hepatotoxic effect or depression of respiration and circulation."[11]

All these things might well have made the difference. Apparently they did. The only large-scale Indian statistics that I could obtain showed astonishing results. They were collected by Arthur Neve, in Kashmir, in 1898. He quoted 78,407 cases of chloroform anaesthesia administered, over the years, in six towns in the sub-Continent. There were only three deaths recorded — a death rate of roughly 1 in 26,000.[12] No hospitals in temperate climates, dealing with Western, or European, patients could produce figures like these. In India, primary cardiac failure was, unwittingly, avoided by the mental attitude of the oriental patients, for in this mode of death mental factors are more important than physical ones.

Only one other point is left for consideration, and that is "delayed chloroform poisoning". Lawrie never mentioned it at all, and may never have seen it or recognised it. Here the dietary factor must have played a part, but luck also stepped in.

Lawrie never really attempted to produce deep anaesthesia with chloroform and so the risk of such after-effects would have been reduced. Indian patients were frequently removed from the hospitals and taken home very soon after operation, and this habit would have tended to conceal deaths due to delayed poisoning, the symptoms of which did not usually begin until two or three days after the anaesthetic. Another factor was the necessity, in India, for burial soon after death; post-mortem examinations were not likely to have been performed in that climate (of weather and of opinion) with any undue frequency.

So there are sound reasons why the dangerous side effects of chloroform — which Lawrie either refused to recognise or was not aware of — should have been encountered so rarely in India, but quite frequently in other places.

237

Lawrie compared his own statistics with those compiled by Roger Williams from the records of St. Bartholomew's Hospital in London.[13,14] Bart's at first sight showed up badly in comparison with Hyderabad but there is a material point which has escaped notice by both sides in this part of the argument. These statistics were collected at a time when major abdominal surgery was very much on the increase. This increase in the scope of surgery, and in operative severity, was likely to be reflected in an increased death rate in the operating theatres and surgical wards of a London teaching hospital, but was far less likely to affect practice in Hyderabad, where most of the surgery was done by one man who had many other responsibilities. The number of abdominal operations performed at the Afzulgunj Hospital, near Hyderabad, must have been quite small. In the journals Lawrie described a total of 18 cases, only one of which, a hysterectomy, was an abdominal procedure; the surgery lasted one hour and a half. In his table of operations for one month (which comprised a very respectable total of 221 in 30 days) the average duration of the operations was just over 12 minutes;[15] so there cannot have been many laparotomies amongst them.

Such as it might have been, the fancied superiority of Hyderabad over a big London teaching hospital was marred by the fact that Lawrie quoted his adversary's figures incorrectly. The mortality rate for ether was 1 in 4,860 and not 1 in 2,754 as quoted by Lawrie. Roger Williams was quick to point out Lawrie's error.[16] Carelessness of this kind creates a doubt, not about Lawrie's honesty, but as to his reliability with figures of any sort.

In mid-1890 a carefully reasoned critique of the Second Hyderabad Commission's Report was published in the *British Medical Journal*. The authors, who had ten years earlier taken part in the investigation organised by the British Medical Association into the safety of chloroform, stated:

"As a matter of common prudence, and especially seeing that when respiration fails we can employ artificial means for its restoration, while if the heart fails, little or nothing can be done to avert a fatal issue, it is incumbent on every one giving chloroform to watch both the pulse and the breathing."[17]

To this rebuke, Lawrie made an excellent, logical reply.

"If this statement is to be acted upon, it is incumbent on everyone giving chloroform to watch the pulse for heart failure, in spite of the fact recorded by the committee themselves that 'if the heart fails, little or nothing can be done to avert a fatal issue'. No teaching could possibly be more dangerous."[18]

In 1894, Dr. Le Cronier Lancaster, of Swansea, described an episode which he considered made a nonsense of Lawrie's beliefs.

"A female aged thirty-seven was given chloroform to facilitate the reduction of a dislocation of the shoulder of over two days' standing. The heart sounds were normal. The chloroform was given on an ordinary wire mask covered with flannel. For about thirty seconds the patient breathed naturally, though somewhat rapidly; there then ensued a short and not severe struggling stage, during which the administration was slackened; she then sank gently back upon the pillow, breathing quietly and deeply. In a few seconds more the breathing ceased with *absolute suddenness*. The pulse was then found to be absent, nor could the heart sounds be heard. The respiration had been in no wise interfered with; the woman was in bed loosely dressed; she had no false teeth, nor had she vomited, nor had the tongue fallen back against the palate. Artificial respiration carried on for over half an hour, the injection of alcohol, and inversion were all useless. The woman had died suddenly. To show how carefully the breathing had been watched, I may say that in discussing the matter afterwards with my surgical colleague I had to ask him whether or not he had commenced any attempts at reduction; as he had merely lifted the arm once and slightly rotated it I do not think that death was caused by shock from pain due to imperfect anaesthesia."[19]

Lawrie never replied to this letter; after all, there really was no reply he could have made. He could, conceivably, have criticised the administration because the anaesthetic was only "slackened" and not stopped altogether during the struggling stage but, at this date, his own practice was similar. He did not introduce his absolute rule of stopping the anaesthetic during struggling until after one of his own patients had died on the table five years later.[20] Before this happened the students at Hyderabad were allowed to slacken or discontinue the anaesthetic as they pleased if the patient struggled. Lawrie could not have complained that the Hyderabad cap had not been used, as he had said that the apparatus was of no importance as long as it allowed plenty of air to be inhaled, and was simple enough not to distract the chloroformist's attention. Nothing could have been simpler than a wire mask.

Again, Lawrie made a perfectly reasonable point when he asked.

"Why are we to continue to study only the experience of those surgeons who cannot give chloroform safely? Why does not *The Lancet* ask the men who do not have deaths to give us their experience for a change?"[21]

This was said during a lecture at the Afzulgunj Hospital but Lawrie, justifiably, hoped that his words would reach a much wider audience of surgeons and chloroformists. In the course of his lecture he had referred to various accounts of fatalities under chloroform and dismissed them all by saying "The reports of chloroform deaths are utterly worthless and unreliable." Such a general, *ex cathedra* condemnation of everybody else's evidence did nothing to strengthen his own argument, especially when no testimony was produced to support his view. Lawrie did not say why he thought that the evidence of others was unreliable and worthless but that his own was credible. Probably, he had in mind the inevitable scrappiness of some of those reports; this was due to the appalling suddenness of the deaths which made accurate observation and time-keeping difficult or impossible. Many of them were, however, as exact and informative as they could possibly have been under the difficult circumstances. In any case, Lawrie's own elaborate, meticulous time-keeping system failed during an emergency which happened as one of his students was giving chloroform to a child. The patient survived, but the account relates that

"The respirations became stertorous, then shallow, then stopped altogether, and no heart sounds could be heard for some time. . . . The notebook was now inadvertently handed over to a student who was not accustomed to take notes, the regular note-taker being absent, and no further entry was made till the conclusion of the operation."[22]

This disregard which Lawrie had for the evidence of other men was due to his fixed idea that sudden death from chloroform, itself, could not occur — that overdosage and gradual failure of respiration during increasingly, and unnecessarily, deep anaesthesia was the only danger. He could only have continued to hold his opinions, as he certainly did, by ignoring or refuting the mounting tide of facts which contradicted them. His beliefs were so deeply ingrained in him that he was prepared to do even this, which is the ultimate heresy of science.

In 1894, Lawrie demonstrated his methods at The London Hospital, in Whitechapel. In his lecture which preceded this demonstration he referred to the setting up of the Second Hyderabad Chloroform Commission.

"I agreed in 1889, and I understood at the time that the rest of the profession agreed, to stand or fall, as regards the action of chloroform on the heart, by the results of the Commission's experiments. The only reservation I made was that nothing the Commission could discover would persuade me that I could not give chloroform safely."[23]

Lawrie could, indeed, give chloroform safely, and he did so for many, many years. Clearly, not everyone could do this but the Commission's findings coupled with Lawrie's unremitting and fervent insistence that it could be given without risk led to the continuance of chloroform's use long after it should, with reason, have been dubbed an unsafe anaesthetic.

There, at The London in 1894, Lawrie admitted publicly that nothing, not even his beloved Commission, could or would be allowed to disturb or

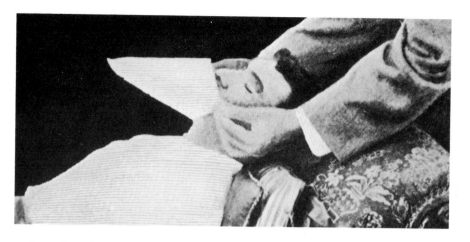

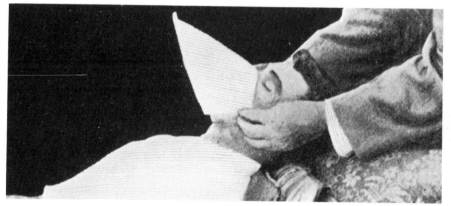

FIGURE 76

The Hyderabad chloroform cap in use.

"As good a form of inhaler as any other is the cloth cone or cap, with a little absorbent cotton stitched into the apex, which is used in Hyderabad. A drachm of chloroform is poured in the cap every three-quarters of a minute or minute, and the cap should be held loosely but closely over the mouth and nose."

The upper picture shows how the administration of chloroform was commenced by covering the mouth and then the nose gently with the cap. The lower illustration depicts how the anaesthesia was maintained with chloroform, air being let in from below.

(Lawrie, E. (1901) *Chloroform: a manual for students and practitioners.* London: Churchill.)

eradicate his fundamental beliefs. This shows a most serious flaw in his scientific attitude, and prevents him from being taken seriously as an investigator. All this in spite of his persistence, his burning enthusiasm, and his own excellent record.

REFERENCES

[1] Lawrie, E. (1901) *Chloroform: a manual for students and practitioners.* London: Churchill.

[2] Clover, T. J. (1871) Chloroform accidents. *British Medical Journal,* **2**, 33–34.

[3] Anonymous (1894) Royal Medical and Surgical Society. *Lancet,* **2**, 23–27.

[4] Silk, J. F. W. (1894) The Hyderabad Chloroform Commission: a criticism of its methods and results. *Lancet,* **2**, 134–135.

[5] Annotation (1892) Chloroform in India and Europe. *British Medical Journal,* **1**, 296.

[6] Neve, A. (1890) Chloroform versus ether. *British Medical Journal,* **1**, 293.

[7] Smyth, J. (1895)*

[8] An Indian Chloroformist. (1894) The Hyderabad experiments and their teaching. *Lancet,* **1**, 1090–1091.

[9] Hill, L. (1897) The causation of chloroform syncope. *British Medical Journal,* **2**, 312–313.

[10] South India. (1892) An accident under chloroform. *Lancet,* **2**, 1199–1200.

[11] Madan, K. E. (1944) Chloroform in India. *British Medical Journal,* **2**, 191–192.

[12] Neve, A. (1898) Chloroform in India. *British Medical Journal,* **2**, 1418–1420.

[13] Lawrie, E. (1891) Chloroform or ether? *British Medical Journal,* **1**, 1280–1281.

[14] Williams, W. R. (1890) The relative safety of anaesthetics. *Lancet,* **1**, 317.

[15] Lawrie, E. (1898) The production of chloroform anaesthesia. *Lancet,* **1**, 1681.

[16] Williams, W. R. (1891) Chloroform or ether? *British Medical Journal,* **1**, 1356.

[17] McKendrick, J. G., Coats, J. & Newman, D. (1890) Remarks on the Report of the Second Hyderabad Chloroform Commission. *British Medical Journal,* **1**, 1345–1349.

[18] Lawrie, E. (1890) The Hyderabad Chloroform Commission. *Lancet,* **1**, 1389–1393.

[19] Le Cronier Lancaster, E. (1894) The Hyderabad Commission and a recent death under chloroform. *Lancet,* **2**, 822.

[20] Lawrie, E. (1901) *Chloroform: A manual for students and practitioners.* London: Churchill.

[21] Lawrie, E. (1892) Clinical lecture on the Hyderabad Chloroform Commission and Professor Wood's address on anaesthesia at Berlin. *Lancet,* **2**, 1143–1145.

[22] Lawrie, E. (1892) Cases of normal chloroform anaesthesia with a note of an accident from abnormal anaesthesia. *British Medical Journal,* **1**, 11–13.

[23] Lawrie, E. (1894) Demonstration of the Hyderabad method of chloroform administration at The London Hospital, May 25th, 1894, *Lancet,* **1**, 1395–1396.

*Editorial footnote:—
Of all Dr. Sykes' references that I wished to quote this was the only one for which I could not find an original and complete text. There is however, no reason to doubt the accuracy of Dr. Sykes' transcription of Dr. Smyth's opinion.

CHAPTER 19

THE WEAK POINTS IN LAWRIE'S CASE

These can be discussed under a fair number of headings, and, although I do not much like this style, I can think of no convenient alternative to writing this part of the story in this fashion.

1. *Lawrie's erroneous, basic assumptions*

There were two of these. Firstly, Syme's dogma of perfect safety, in which Lawrie believed so fervently, was founded upon a personal experience far too small to support the vast superstructure which was built upon it. Secondly, this dogma depended to a large extent on a spurious argument. By 1855, the year of Syme's lecture, thirteen deaths from chloroform had occurred in London, but there had been only one in Edinburgh. Syme, therefore, assumed that the Edinburgh method was far safer than that used in London. He ignored the fact that London was thirteen times as large as Edinburgh; this figure was just as available to Syme, from the Census figures of the day, as they were to me one hundred years later.[1] The statistical significance is obvious.

Syme's erroneous, indestructible — but dangerous — doctrine lingered on for many years. Its adherents were not at all half-hearted in their blind, unreasoning and unreasonable faith. No theological belief could have been held and defended with greater vigour and intolerance. The difference, unfortunately, was that the defence of religious beliefs sometimes led to the deaths of the believers, but the defence of this, medical, creed not infrequently led to the deaths of other, innocent people.

Some figures were published in 1931 which dealt a final and shattering blow to those still with a lingering belief in the safety of chloroform in Scotland and elsewhere. The statistics were from Scottish sources and from Scottish authors, so there can be no question of racial, antichloroform bias. The argument was as follows. In 1927 there were 103 anaesthetic deaths in Scotland and 596 in England and Wales. No attempt was made by the authors to correlate these with the countries' populations. These, as recorded in the nearest Census (conducted in 1931), showed that the population of Scotland and of England and Wales bore a ratio of 1 to 8·24. So there should have been more than eight times as many deaths in England and Wales than in Scotland. The actual figure was just 5·8 times as many. Put another way, if the death rates had been exactly equal, England and Wales would have suffered 848 deaths compared to the 103 in Scotland — that is 252 more than actually occurred. This argument hardly lends support to the earlier, contemptuous dismissal of anaesthesia and its teaching south of the Scottish border. I have no doubt that earlier, detailed figures would reveal the same pattern.

Further condemnation of chloroform's alleged safety in Scotland was supplied by Frederic Hewitt in 1901.

"I may, however, refer to a somewhat interesting incident bearing upon the supposed safety of chloroform in the country north of the Tweed. A few years ago I had the honour to receive a deputation from an important Scotch hospital in which, so far as my memory serves me, no less than nine chloroform accidents had occurred in one year. I was asked to express an opinion as to the best form of ether inhaler."[2]

In spite of all the opposition Lawrie was still claiming absolute safety for chloroform in 1914, less than a year before his death.

"Ever since chloroform was discovered by the late Sir James Simpson there have been two distinct schools of anaesthesia, which, for convenience, we may still call the Edinburgh and the London schools. The Edinburgh school, represented by Professor Syme, watched the breathing alone for the effect of the anaesthetic — 'you never see anyone here with his finger on the pulse while chloroform is given' — the London school watched the breathing and the pulse as well.

"At first sight it might appear that the anaesthetist who watches the pulse as well as the breathing is doing more for the safety of his patient than he who watches the respiration alone. This, however, is not the case. The anaesthetist who watches the pulse for the effect of chloroform is doing the one thing which makes the administration dangerous, and which must make a certain percentage of deaths inevitable. . . . The first sign of heart failure given by the pulse would merely indicate . . . that the breathing had stopped some time before, and every case would die. In the second place, clinically, to prevent the inhalation of an overdose and to keep the heart intact during anaesthesia, the whole of the chloroformist's undivided attention must be concentrated on the patient's breathing-"[3]

2. A distinction without a difference

Syme extolled the importance of his "principles" as opposed to the London "rules", and this supposed difference was stressed by Lawrie *ad nauseam*. He seemed to think that there was some special and mystical virtue in a few simple rules so long as they were referred to as principles. Syme's method was, actually, the crudest rule of thumb imaginable — an elementary way of doing something which he considered to be of very slight importance, and which, anyway, could be explained in ten minutes.

3. Alterations in the unalterable

Syme did not always adhere strictly to his own "principles" even though, to Lawrie, they were immutable. But not to Syme himself. Dr. Robert Farquharson wrote:

"In the palmy days of Edinburgh, when that great surgeon reigned supreme, I had the honour to be his dresser, and afterwards his 'supernumerary', and therefore had the opportunity not only of watching his methods, but of helping to maintain the anaesthesia when the house-surgeon was otherwise engaged.

"We all remember how rough and ready the process was — an unstinted and unmeasured quantity of Duncan and Flockhart's excellent chloroform was poured, not dribbled, onto a towel which was then laid over the patient's face, and when the inevitable struggling began, I well remember how Syme's little hand was firmly pressed over the mouth and nose so as to ensure a rapid lapse into insensibility . . ."[4]

It is impossible to imagine any grosser breach of Syme's most important principle "plenty of air".

4. Bias due to enthusiasm

There can be no doubt that Lawrie was extremely biased in his judgements — more so than can be explained by single-minded enthusiasm. Indeed, the Commission owed its existence solely to Lawrie's enthusiasm for Syme's views and his wish to prove, in the laboratory, what he had himself demonstrated clinically in India.

All enthusiasts tend to be impetuous and impatient and to ignore, or minimise, evidence which conflicts with their own opinions. This impetuosity was shown in the work of the Commission itself which attempted to do too much work in too short a time. The Nizam had been quite prepared to pay for an extension of the Commission's work if more time was needed.[5] Brunton, however, could not have stayed abroad and away from London any longer.[6] After all, he had had many lean years as a physiologist, and was making his career as a consulting physician. He explained that the work of the Commission had been done in a short time, but not in a hurry. Lack of time was the excuse for work which was left undone, not for imperfections in work actually performed. Nonetheless, Brunton completely reversed his previously declared opinion of chloroform's lack of safety in just a handful of weeks, having been caught up in the uncritical enthusiasm of the Hyderabad chloroformists.

5. *The effect of cantharides on the hedgehog — again*

The results of the Commission's animal experiments were transferred to man, and were assumed to be infallible — always a risky thing to do. I pointed out in *Volume One*, cantharides has no effect on the hedgehog, but has a devastating effect on human beings.[1] As George Eastes, of London, put it:

"Surgeon-Major Lawrie considers that 'Syme's principles have stood the test of experience, and been proved by the Hyderabad Commission to rest on a secure physiological foundation'; and that 'Hyderabad students can be taught to give chloroform with guaranteed safety.' Now, so far as the 'test of experience' is concerned, it is indeed remarkable, if not unique, that with his many thousands of cases he himself has never met with a single death. . . . But as to the value of the 'secure physiological foundation' one may be more sceptical. For although the experiments of the Commission were most elaborate and quite worthy of Dr. Lauder Brunton's high reputation, the 'practical conclusions' appended to their report appear to be inconsequent and misguiding. Possibly the one precise lesson that may be drawn from the experiments is 'that chloroform may be given to dogs,' and some other animals, 'by inhalation with perfect safety and without any fear of accidental death, if only the respiration, and nothing but the respiration, is carefully attended to throughout.' But, directly this deduction is extended to the case of human beings — as in the 'practical conclusion' which states that 'the administrator should be guided as to the effect entirely by the respiration,' and that 'his only object, while producing anaesthesia is to see that respiration is not interfered with,' — it meets with the strenuous opposition of the most experienced anaesthetists of the day, who consider it to be very unsafe teaching, . . . therefore, English anaesthetists, after experiments on human beings that amount to many hundreds of thousands . . . reject chloroform on the ground that it is not trustworthy, and advise that it should not be used where ether can be employed. On the other hand, the Commission, after 430 experiments on lower animals, would teach us that chloroform is absolutely safe for human beings, if only certain rules, which many practised anaesthetists deem questionable, be followed during its administration. . . . The most unfavourable statistics respecting chloroform that I have seen — those of Mr. W. Roger Williams . . . give the mortality as 1 in 1,236 administrations. Perhaps if the Commission had performed 1,236 experiments (instead of 430 only) they might have found one animal in whom their usual sequence of events — *viz.*, stoppage of the respiration before cessation of the heart's action — did not occur."[7]

6. A change in the unchangeable

On at least two occasions Lawrie made changes in the method which he had, for years, proclaimed as perfect. In so doing he admitted that either perfection could be improved upon, or that his beloved method had its drawbacks and dangers after all. Now, it is the duty and the glory of Science to change — to alter theories as new facts appear and conflict with them; but it is also the glory of Science to admit its imperfection and to strive for improvement. Once perfection has been claimed change of any sort appears ridiculous.

The first alteration which Lawrie made concerned the depth of anaesthesia which was necessary before surgery could be safely begun. Only twice, in the whole, prolonged controversy is the possibility of early chloroform death mentioned by any of the Hyderabad team. As one of its "Practical Conclusions" the Commission stated

"As a rule, no operation should be commenced until the patient is fully under the influence of the anaesthetic, so as to avoid all chance of death from surgical shock or fright."[8]

Earlier, Lawrie had written a letter to *The Lancet* defending the First Hyderabad Chloroform Commission's Report.

"It is conceivable that syncope may occur in the initial stages of inhalation of chloroform, but in the course of a very large experience I have never met with a single instance of such an accident, and if it ever does occur it cannot be due to chloroform poisoning, though it might be caused by fright or shock."[9]

In his own, numerous, personal writings Lawrie repeatedly denied that this was a possibility at all — in spite of constant reports of such fatalities from all over the world. Deaths from chloroform, he insisted, were always due to overdose.[10] He, also, considered that what *The Lancet* referred to as primary and secondary syncope was nothing more than an effect similar to that of vagal stimulation of the heart with its slowing of the heart rate and fall in blood pressure. This, the Report stated, was actually a safeguard against overdose.

"The failure of the heart, if such it can be called, instead of being a danger to the animal, proved to be a positive safeguard, by preventing the absorption of the residual chloroform and its distribution through the system."[8]

Lawrie, evidently, felt so strongly about not starting the surgery until the patient was completely anaesthetised that, six years later, he abandoned this recommendation of the Commission altogether. He no longer made even a pretence of believing in it, which was surprising in view of his having proclaimed the perfection and infallibility of the Hyderabad method for years, provided that it was rigidly followed in every detail. In 1897 he wrote:

"Until two years ago the rule in the Afzulgunj Hospital was to produce complete anaesthesia with chloroform if the patient desired to have it, in every case, without exception, that was fit for an operation. In a large majority of the cases the operations were of a trifling description and of short or momentary duration, but the Edinburgh doctrine was almost invariably followed, and no operation, however trivial, was performed, or even commenced, before the patient was fully under the influence of the anaesthetic. In this way much valuable time was wasted, and patients who suffered from whitlows, abscesses, fistluae, hydrocoele and the thousand and one conditions which necessitate minor but painful surgical procedures were often incapacitated for a whole day or more afterwards by chloroform sickness or dyspepsia. However, as the Hyderabad Commission has proved that chloroform and shock are incompatibles, and that 'primary chloroform syncope' is a myth, the old prejudice against beginning an operation before the patient is 'over' was finally cast aside in 1895, and since then nearly all minor operations have been performed under partial anaesthesia with chloroform."[11]

Of course, all that the Commission — as distinct from Lawrie, with his own vast clinical experience — was entitled to say was that primary chloroform syncope had not been seen in the five or six hundred animals which they had used. This had no bearing whatever on its incidence in human beings. However, to return to analgesia, or partial anaesthesia:

"In this method the chloroform is administered in drachm doses, poured on the top of the cap at minute intervals until the patient becomes unconscious. The moment consciousness is abolished the incision, or puncture, or whatever it may be, is made. The chloroform is then usually stopped, and the dressings are applied while consciousness is returning. Partial anaesthesia has been employed in this manner in more than 2,000 cases, and it is now established as a routine method of practice . . . it is attended with absolutely no risk."

This last was a rash, and completely unjustifiable statement. Nonetheless, Lawrie continued to use this method of chloroform administration for partial anaesthesia, and wrote other accounts of it.[12, 13] In one of these he wrote "In Hyderabad chloroform is given by students in strict accordance with Syme's principles, the heart is ignored, and we have no deaths."[13] Eleven months later a death occurred in Hyderabad, and, to Lawrie's credit, he faithfully recorded it. The event must have been an appalling shock for him, even though he had been away from his hospital at the time. It was his method which had been used.[14]

Lawrie's plan of partial anaesthesia, or chloroform analgesia, did not die with him. It was still in use many years later and, in 1944, Herbert H. Brown, of Worthing, Sussex advocated it. It was, he said "as I have proved on many occasions . . . quite free from any danger".[14a]

7. Unjustified generalisations

This extract is a fairly typical example of Lawrie's style.

"In England the teaching of anaesthetics is in the hands of professional anaesthetists who 'funk' the heart and deaths from chloroform take place, according to Leonard Hill, by the dozen and, according to Roger Williams, no less than once in every 1,236 inhalations. The deaths under anaesthesia in England represent an appalling picture of the incapacity of the medical profession as regards the administration of these drugs. This incapacity is altogether due to the absolute want of training of English students in the art of chloroform administration on Syme's principles, which have been established on a scientific basis by the Hyderabad Commission."[13]

This was written in 1898. An ill-considered attack like this must count as another weak point in Lawrie's argument. His medical education took place in Edinburgh, and most of his professional life was spent in India. His knowledge of English teaching hospitals and their methods must have been very limited, and gathered by hearsay at that. It is also just possible to recognise here a fragment of Syme's lecture, "all that I would say respecting our brethren in London, is that they have not been so fortunate as to get into the right way in the first instance".

Understandably, there were several vociferous replies to this "grape-shot" method of argument. Frederic Hewitt said of Lawrie's letter that it was "certainly not characterised by moderation in language".[2] Hewitt pointed out that ether (which Lawrie had referred to as a "degrading and throttling thralldom"[14]) had a much wider margin of safety than chloroform, and that this was important because the English surgeons of the time expected "patients to be kept, not, as Colonel Lawrie apparently keeps his patients, *moderately* anaesthetised, but profoundly narcotised . . ." This was said about 20 years after the rise of abdominal surgery, but some 40 years before the relaxant era, so Hewitt's statement was perfectly correct as far as the increasing proportion of cases for which deep anaesthesia was necessary.

Dr. Bellamy Gardner noted that he and his fellow students had, in fact, been thoroughly trained by Dr. Hewitt at the Charing Cross Hospital in London eleven years previously,[15] and Dr. Dudley Buxton noted:

"It is perhaps a pity that before making such a sweeping statement Lieutenant-Colonel Lawrie should not have ascertained what is really taught in London. At University College Hospital the students have actual control of, and responsibility concerning, the patient from the induction to the end of narcosis. I have little doubt a similar course is adopted elsewhere. The period of chloroformist clerkship is one month, which, as Lieutenant-Colonel Lawrie thinks, is more than sufficient for the average student."[16]

Frederic Hewitt again noted:

". . . Lieutenant-Colonel Lawrie fully realises . . . he cannot resist the temptation of continuing his laudable task of collecting and replacing the numerous fragments of the Hyderabad idol. I can only again express my regret that he should persistently obtrude this mending process upon a weary audience. . . . Our requirements are of a totally different order to those which apparently exist in India. . . . Some years ago Lieutenant-Colonel Lawrie came with two assistants to The London Hospital and chloroform was administered in the Hyderabad fashion in two straightforward cases. But the type of anaesthesia produced was distinctly inferior to that which may be witnessed any day of the week in the operating theatres of our hospitals. A case presenting greater scope for skill in anaesthetising was prepared for Lieutenant-Colonel Lawrie at University College Hospital, but although the theatre was crowded in expectation of his arrival he failed to put in an appearance.

"Interesting as this correspondence has been, I fear I must decline to continue it further, for I cannot conceive that any useful purpose can be served by discussing such inconvenient and obsolete means of anaesthetisation as those advocated by Lieutenant-Colonel Lawrie."[17]

The demonstration at The London Hospital, to which Hewitt referred, took place on May 25th, 1894, at the invitation of Mr. Frederick Treves. Lawrie preceded his demonstration by delivering a most patronising lecture which concluded by exhorting his audience:

". . . to abandon the firm conviction that chloroform acts directly upon the heart and to completely alter your principles of chloroformisation; but the men of 'The London' with such a surgeon as Mr. Treves at their head, seconded by a man the calibre of Dr. Hewitt, are not the men I take them to be if they do not conquer this difficulty and bring the question of the administration of chloroform, in the solution of which we in India have played a humble and up to now a distant part, to a successful issue."[18]

The two cases, one an appendicectomy and the other a nephrectomy, were anaesthetised by one of Lawrie's assistants, Dr. Mahomed Abdul Ghany who used a Hyderabad chloroform cap. In both cases "there was occasional rigidity of the abdominal muscles, which interfered with the surgeon's manipulations. Lawrie attributed this to his assistant's not being used to Treves' method of operating: Treves declared himself satisfied by the Hyderabad method, and the only objection he had had to make was that the abdominal muscles were not completely relaxed."

8. The second improvement upon perfection

The second important modification which Lawrie made in order to perfect his avowedly perfect method was noticed by Dr. Bellamy Gardner in 1901.

"'Hyderabad methods' of inducing chloroform narcosis seem to have undergone a radical change since March 20th, 1899, when, according to Lieutenant-Colonel Lawrie's book on Chloroform, a death took place during the struggling stage of anaesthesia and he laid down the law 'never to give chloroform while there is struggling and irregular breathing.' 'Formerly' — i.e., previously to this date — he says, 'there was always an element of chance, and, consequently, of risk in the administration.' 'Hyderabad methods,' then, were not so perfect from 1892 to 1899 . . ."[15]

Rather hard on Lawrie, perhaps, but he certainly had asked for it. It is not at all surprising that the London anaesthetists were, at long last, becoming a little tired of being told by Lawrie how incompetent they were. Lawrie, himself, said:

"The introduction of the rule never to give chloroform while there is struggling and irregular breathing has already been followed by a considerable improvement in clinical results. Formerly there was always an element of chance and consequently of risk in the administration, shown in the cases of accidental overdosing which from time to time occurred: now overdosing never takes place."[14]

9. Misstatements

Note the date of the Hyderabad chloroform death — March, 1899 — because eight and a half years after this Lawrie, referring yet again to Syme's principles, wrote:

". . . the fact remains that if chloroform is given on these principles, brought to perfection as they have been by the brilliant work of Sir Lauder Brunton and Surgeon-General Bomford on the Hyderabad Commission, danger and death are alike impossible."[19]

In short, the Commission brought the whole matter to absolute perfection in 1889, but in 1899 a serious and fatal defect in the method was discovered. Death was impossible — but a death had occurred.

Lawrie cannot be criticised for his one fatality; rather, he should be praised for his outstandingly successful record. But he must be criticised for making such an illogical statement as this.

If we accept his figures as correct (and I believe they are accurate) Lawrie was quite entitled to claim for himself an unparalleled and amazing success rate. From 1892 to 1900 he gave, or supervised, 17,300 anaesthetics with only one death. If we add to this figure a realistic proportion of his other cases dealt with in the twenty years before he began to keep careful anaesthetic records (his figure of "forty or fifty thousand" was undoubtedly an exaggeration) we can safely conclude that no other person has ever approached this achievement. Lawrie was entitled to claim great safety, but no more. To have suggested that his, or any other, method could never have been fatal was to reduce the meaning of his words to mere sounds without significance. Further, he made this outrageous suggestion after a death at Hyderabad when his own method had been used.

Lawrie's intransigent and truculent manner, combined with his inaccuracy for detail combine to weaken his whole case. His habit of treating other men, of great experience, wisdom and skill, as though they were incompetent and foolish when coupled with his own devastating certainty that he, alone, understood the truth of things, was certain to have antagonised his opponents. Historians, likewise, are unlikely to be taken in by his filibustering.

10. Contradictions

On occasions Lawrie contradicted himself. This is not, really, surprising in such a long and complicated controversy which lasted for some 26 years — from 1889 until his death in 1915. In a letter written in 1907, Lawrie said

"If cardiac syncope were . . . the principal danger of anaesthesia, it would be imperative to watch the pulse while chloroform is given. But . . . watching the pulse means death under chloroform, because stoppage of the heart is its final effect. Cardiac syncope from chloroform, therefore, can only be the final sign of fatal overdosing."[20]

If this was true, what should become of Lawrie's argument based on the discovery made by the Commission that the cardiac inhibition caused by vagal stimulation was actually a safeguard, since it caused less chloroform to be removed from the lungs and conveyed to the vital centres by the blood stream? Besides, Lawrie overlooked the fact that the Hyderabad Commission never investigated primary syncope at all. It was only concerned with overdosage, and its results. The deaths which occurred during the induction of anaesthesia for the experiments were ignored.

11. Contraventions of the Commission's directive

The Report of the Commission records the usual methods of anaesthesia used by the experimenters.

"For experiments on the general action of chloroform the animal was usually placed upon a table and held by several assistants. An inhaler, consisting of a conical bag of cloth containing a sponge or absorbent cotton-wool with the anaesthetic, was then placed over the animal's mouth and nostrils, and kept there as long as necessary. While one observer watched for the loss of reflex from the cornea, the cessation of respiration, stoppage of the pulse, and arrest of the heart, another seated at an adjoining table with a watch before him noted down the times at which each event occurred. The corneal reflex was ascertained by simply touching the cornea with a finger or a blunt instrument, such as the point of an aneurysm needle. The cessation of breathing was ascertained by simple ocular inspection of the thorax and diaphragm, the presence or absence of the pulse by feeling the femoral artery with the finger, and the entire stoppage of the heart's action by watching the movements of a needle pushed through the thoracic walls into the heart. The movements of this needle were rendered more evident by a straw bearing a small paper flag being fixed to the end which projected outside the thorax. Animals anaesthetised by this method struggled while they were held until the anaesthetic had had time to take effect. In order to avoid struggling another method was adopted. This consisted in simply lifting the animal into a wooden box 3 ft. 10 in. long by 1 ft. 5 in. broad, and 1 ft. 7 in. deep, and putting on the lid, in which there was an opening. Through this opening was passed a large piece of blotting-paper on which half an ounce or more of chloroform had been poured. A piece of wood or glass was then placed over the opening in the lid, and in a short time the anaesthetic took effect. To prevent too large admixture of air a strip of spongio-piline was nailed round the edges of the box and covered with vaseline, so that the lid shut down air-tight. Even when a piece of wood was used to close the aperture in the lid at first it was usually replaced by glass, when the chloroform began to take effect, as the movements of the animal could thus be watched. When it fell down insensible it was usually taken out at once, and if prolonged anaesthesia was required, as for blood-pressure experiments, an additional quantity of anaesthetic was administered on a cap."[21]

Lawrie's original directive to the First Commission insisted that the chloroform should be given to the animals in just the same way as it was administered to the patients at the Afzalgunj and Residency Hospitals in Hyderabad. Clearly, with the use of the box, the instruction was frequently disregarded as far as the induction — arguably the most interesting, dangerous and relevant stage — was concerned.

12. Important evidence overlooked

It is clear from the Report that deaths in the induction box occurred quite frequently. There were no less than nine of these in a series of 154 experiments — an incidence of almost six per cent. This, it must be remembered, in the course of a work which was designed to prove the absolute safety of chloroform anaesthesia! Lauder Brunton spoke of these deaths at a meeting in London soon after his return from Hyderabad.

"The most important experiments that we did were our accidental deaths. We had a large proportion of them, much larger than ordinary surgeons have, and we could always trace the mode in which they occurred. We knew that the time of day had something to do with it. The deaths did not occur in the morning when everyone was looking sharply after things, when we were not hurried, when there was plenty of time, but they occurred in the middle of the day when we resumed our experiments after the interval for lunch. An experiment was finished before lunch, then there was an interval, during which we left the apparatus standing, but the drums had to be blackened, and a lot of little odds and ends had to be done. We did not want to lose time, and while things were being got ready, some one would put the animal under chloroform. The way in which it was done was this: we simply had a big packing case into which we popped the dog, and put in some chloroform on blotting paper; after a time the animal quietly went over, and then he was taken out. Someone looked in perhaps just to see that he was thoroughly over, and if he was not we gave him a little more time, put him back in the box, and put in a little more chloroform. Then, instead of watching, the man attending to the case would go away to black a drum, and when he went back he found the dog was dead. Another thing which is very instructive is the fact that very few deaths occurred upon the table. When a man was giving chloroform who was accustomed to give it at a hospital very few deaths occurred. But one day he was too much intent upon the operation; he had not seen it done before, and instead of watching the animal as he ought to have done, he was watching the other man operate, and the first thing that was noticed by a third person present who was standing by, was that the animal was not breathing. The animal indeed was already dead. Another case of accidental death occurred to myself. I was doing two things at once, giving chloroform and putting a cannula into the trachea. It was a peculiarly-shaped T-tube that I was putting in. Another man was doing the same thing at the same time, and I am sorry to say that we were running a race; I was trying to get my tube in before him, and he was trying to get his in before me, and in doing the thing as quickly as I could I forgot to attend to the respiration of the monkey, and he died. It was simply for the want of attention to the respiration."[22]

Brunton said that these deaths were important. They would have been if anybody had bothered to investigate them properly, but no attempt was made to find out whether the heart or the breathing had stopped first. Lawrie, in 1894, also referred to the deaths in the induction box.

"The fatal result was brought about either by neglecting to watch the condition of the respiration during or after the administration of chloroform, especially while the carotid artery was being exposed, or from a rapid administration of chloroform in the endeavour to prevent or check struggles. In all the cases of accidental death the usual chloroformist was absent, and no one was attending to the chloroform. The notes would have been more complete if someone could have watched the condition of the animal, and noted the gradual but unheeded cessation of respiration without calling attention to it. As it is one has to be content with the remark that the breathing was noticed to have stopped at some particular time, but there is nothing to throw any light upon the conditions during the important period that immediately preceded this discovery."[23]

This is an amazing assumption, that death was due to respiratory failure. Nobody can be surprised that Lawrie believed in its accuracy, but Brunton's uncritical acceptance of the notion is impossible to explain satisfactorily. There was no evidence whatsoever to support the idea since no one had made any observations of the animals at the time of death. In any case, why were the animals not watched; money was no object, and extra observers could have been recruited with ease. Instead the fatalities were facilely explained away on the basis of Lawrie's preconceived ideas to which Brunton, lamely, subscribed. Syme — and Lawrie — had both said that the pulse could not stop before respiration, and so there appeared to the Commission no point at all in pursuing the induction deaths any further.

In the hospital practice four people, usually students, were needed to give chloroform by the Hyderabad method. One held the chloroform cap, another measured out the doses of chloroform, a third took careful notes and a fourth acted as timekeeper. Clearly this was not always done in the laboratory experiments, and this is, again, at odds with Lawrie's original directive.

13. Only one-third of the problem was investigated

Lawrie denied the existence of primary cardiac failure due to chloroform, and the Commission did not conscientiously examine this important, possible cause of death at all. It therefore ignored one third of the whole question of chloroform's dangers. The Commission was, by and large, preoccupied with the problem of overdosage and of how that could be avoided. The third, major problem with chloroform — that of delayed chloroform poisoning — was never even cited. Admittedly, this had only really been mentioned for the first time in a British journal in 1888,[24] and it was not until 1894 that Leonard Guthrie had really publicised the subject,[25, 26] Nonetheless, it is extraordinary that this rare, but dangerous, complication was never mentioned during the controversy by either side, even after 1894 when ether became increasingly popular as attempts were made to avoid the inescapable dangers of chloroform.

One thing quite clear from the Commission's Report is that the members did not know, at all, how to use ether and did not trouble to learn. (In the Report itself it is stated that 109 pints of chloroform were used, as were 11 pints of ether. Making allowance for the eight to one relative potency of these two drugs, it is reasonable to say that ether must have been used in just over one per cent. of the Commission's experiments. So they did not get much practice.)

By and large, most anaesthetists at that time were not so much concerned with the problem of chloroform overdose which could be minimised by skill, constant practice and experience. Instead they were worried about the two dangers which Lawrie never mentioned at all — primary cardiac failure, and delayed chloroform poisoning — and which were seemingly unpredictable, unpreventable, and fatal. I can find no evidence that Edward Lawrie was ever coaxed into print on the subject of delayed chloroform poisoning.

14. Reckless statements

Some of Lawrie's remarks were, indeed, surprising. In one of his more vitriolic replies to Dr. Dudley Buxton, of University College Hospital, London, who was one of Lawrie's most persistent critics, he really let himself go. This was in 1914.

"It is amusing that Dr. Buxton should suddenly profess himself to be an 'enthusiastic admirer of my splendid work and valuable book', seeing that for the last five-and-twenty years he has assailed the work of the Hyderabad Commission with every possible kind of detraction and misstatement . . . an essential feature of his plan of giving chloroform is 'to keep a finger upon an artery' . . . this is, as I have repeatedly insisted, a thoroughly dangerous way of giving chloroform. . . . The failure of the heart which may occur under Dr. Buxton's plan of giving chloroform is a positive sign of maladministration."[27]

These words were addressed publicly, not to a stupid and backward junior student, but to a senior consultant anaesthetist who had, at that time, given anaesthetics for 29 years. They could, with advantage, have been phrased somewhat differently. Buxton believed that it was always important to feel the pulse since signs of its weakening indicated overdosage. Of this view Lawrie wrote:

"The dosage of chloroform is a point of absolutely no importance, and in whatever way the drug is given it must always be a matter of guesswork."

By 1914 there were several accurate vapourisers for chloroform, but these Lawrie chose to ignore in favour of his simple, inaccurate chloroform cap. Lawrie's reply to Buxton concluded:

"In taking leave of this subject for the present, I venture to submit that the question of surgical anaesthesia cannot be settled by controversy. It is not a personal matter, but is one of such enormous importance to our profession and the public that it demands — most urgently — a full and searching examination by the British Medical Association. I plead guilty to being under the influence of the *idée fixe*; it is that deaths under anaesthesia are, practically, all preventable, and I feel sure that they would cease if the inquiry which I suggest were made."

Amazing! Without moving, intellectually, one single inch Lawrie had come full circle. Twenty-four years earlier he had written, of the First Hyderabad Chloroform Commission:

"Chloroform administration constitutes, in my humble opinion, the most pressing and important question in the whole range of practical surgery; and if *The Lancet* will not accept the conclusions of the Hyderabad Commission, it is incumbent on it to urge the appointment of a ... Commission, composed of men of wide experience in chloroform, to confirm or disprove them."[9]

In 1903, Lawrie wrote to the *British Medical Journal* to complain that:

"It is a reproach to British science and surgery that my work should be ignored, and that there should still be two distinct and irreconcilable methods of chloroform administration. In the one, which is founded, on pseudo-scientific experimental data and antiquated beliefs, the heart is dragged in as a factor, while in my method, which is founded on proved facts — experimental and clinical — the heart is completely ignored. In the former fright of the heart predominates, and deaths are unavoidable; in the latter there is no fear but that of overdosing, and deaths are impossible."[28]

This was written just four years after the death on the table at Hyderabad, and was clearly untrue. Besides, how could Lawrie have referred to the fear of overdosage on one occasion, and on another have said that the dose of chloroform was of absolutely no importance?

Whether Lawrie's reckless statements had any harmful effects is impossible to say, or to prove, but at least one anaesthetist in London thought that the Commission's claims for the absolute safety of chloroform were factors in the, then, increasing death rate during anaesthesia and surgery. Dr. J. F. W. Silk said that "The great increase of deaths under chloroform had taken place mainly since the promulgation of the results arrived at by the Hyderabad Commission."[23] We would do well to remember that, at the time of Dr. Silk's observation, the scope of surgery was expanding rapidly and this fact, too, could be expected to increase mortality during surgery, irrespective of the anaesthetic involved.

15. Lawrie's method in other hands and other lands

Dr. Cecil Leaf, who spent a while in Hyderabad, wrote an impassioned defence of Lawrie's methods in 1892,[29] and in the following year sent *The Lancet* a résumeé of experiments on chloroform which he had carried out in Hyderabad together with a 200 page volume of his results.[30] He adduced no new evidence and relied on the old arguments. He, like his predecessors, anaesthetised most of his animals in an induction box, but he did not study the induction period at all. However, he concluded that his results, as far as they went, were in accordance with those of the Hyderabad Commission. Having done all this work, and studied with Lawrie in Hyderabad Dr. Leaf, if anyone, should have known the proper way to give chloroform with perfect safety. Not so; later in 1893 he had to report a death under chloroform anaesthesia, administered by himself, at The London Hospital.[31]

16. Total neglect of the pulse — the one safeguard?

Professor W. A. Stevenson of the Army Medical School at Netley, wrote of two cases which made a nonsense of Lawrie's insistence that it was dangerous to feel the pulse during chloroform anaesthesia.

"One was the case of a child aged three years, on whom the operation of needling was being performed for a congenital cataract; but as the operation was completed the boy's face suddenly became pale, and the pulse was found to be imperceptible at the wrist and in the neck. At this time no cessation of the movements of the chest and abdominal walls took place, and air was heard to pass in and out of the lungs freely. Under the use of the interrupted current, friction and ether subcutaneously, the attack of syncope passed off. The second case was that of a man on whom the 'radical cure' was being performed for an inguinal hernia. The patient took the chloroform perfectly until the sac of the hernia was twisted. When this was done the man's face immediately blanched and the pulse became imperceptible, whilst the movements of respiration continued vigorous and effective. Ether was injected, the head lowered, sponges wrung out of very hot water were applied over the heart, and electricity to the neck. In about five minutes the pulse was again to be felt and the man recovered. Had the rules laid down by the Hyderabad Commission for the administration of chloroform been carried out in these two cases, had the indications afforded by observation of the pulse been disregarded and the condition of the respiration alone noted, the chances are that the deaths of these patients would have had to be added to the already too long list of 'deaths under chloroform.' But, luckily the cessation of the pulse was one of the danger signals which was being looked for, and on its appearance steps were immediately taken to prevent the catastrophe of which it was the first sign."[32]

Joseph Mills, the Administrator of Anaesthetics at St. Bartholomew's Hospital, London had, in 1880, been of the same opinion.

"During the present year I have given anaesthetics at St. Bartholomew's Hospital 1,420 times, and of these chloroform 572 times; and in three of these cases I have had reason to be thankful that I carefully watched the pulse during the administration. I believe that had I not done so I should have lost the patients."[33]

Each of these three cases recovered; in all, Mills was able to quote six such cases in his series of 9,000 patients to whom he had given anaesthetics.

17. Physiological criticisms

There were many of these, and a great number were as outspoken as Lawrie had been himself. In 1897, Leonard Hill, who was Lecturer in Physiology at The London Hospital, gave a long and detailed address before The Society of Anaesthetists on "The Causation of Chloroform Syncope".

"The whole endeavour of this paper is directed towards the establishment of the true pathological cause of chloroform syncope, and the controversion of one of the most pernicious and dangerous doctrines ever put before the medical profession. This doctrine, so long received by many with credence, is that chloroform kills by paralysing the respiratory centre. Supported by the wealth of the Hyderabad Government, furthered by the prejudiced enthusiasm of Surgeon-Lieutenant-Colonel Lawrie, this statement, upheld by a series of experiments, many so careless in execution that they could not for one moment be accepted by a trained physiologist — this doctrine that the paralysis of the respiratory centre causes chloroform syncope, has been industriously spread abroad, and instilled into the minds of the whole medical world.

"Chloroform syncope is a subject on which every medical man must have more or less clinical experience. It is one, therefore, that naturally each feels qualified to discuss or to write about in the medical journals. What is wanted at their hands is a careful record of the symptoms observed in chloroform syncope, rather than an addition to the mass of literature dealing with the theory of the subject. . . . In a certain institution in Great Britain, in the course of a recent year, there were out of some three or four thousand administrations no fewer than twelve fatalities. This is no exceptional case. The deaths from chloroform are not recorded in the medical journals, for these reflect upon the reputation of the administrator and the institution in which they occur. . . . In my discussion of the subject I shall confine myself purely to the experimental side of the question. . . . The point to consider is whether these experiments are done by competent and trained enquirers."[34]

Referring to the accidental, and unobserved deaths of almost six per cent. of the Commission's experimental animals, Leonard Hill wrote:

"In this . . . the Commission gives away their whole case. They never observed these accidental deaths; they left the primary anaesthetisation to the hands of somebody who was not the usual chloroformist, and may have been the laboratory servant. In all cases of chloroform syncope occurring during primary anaesthetisation I have carefully observed the symptoms. Either the pulse ceases before the respiration or the two cease together. . . . On rapidly opening the thoracic cavity I have always found the heart to be . . . in a state of paralytic dilatation. The cardiac musculature of the heart may rhythmically twitch but entirely fails to empty its cavities. . . .

"Not only the work of all physiologists, but also the tracings of the Commission, when rightly interpreted, prove that paralysis of the circulatory mechanism, and not of the respiratory centre, is to be dreaded by the anaesthetist."

Although Hill had not mentioned him by name, this was a swingeing attack on Lauder Brunton as well as on the Commission as a whole. Brunton made no comment, but Lawrie wrote a long reply to the criticism. His most interesting point was:

"What Mr. Leonard Hill means by stating that the Hyderabad Commission have given themselves away in the matter of the accidental deaths it is not possible to imagine. The accidental deaths which took place during the research of the Hyderabad Commission were published to show that there was no truth in the idea that there is something in the climate of India which prevents accidents from chloroform. The Hyderabad Commission never pretended to draw any scientific value from them as to the exact cause of the accidents, the circumstances under which they occurred making that impossible. Mr. Leonard Hill, on the other hand, just like the clinical accident-producing chloroformist, wants to persuade us that there was evidence of paralysis of the heart in similar cases which happened in his hands. This is exactly what the Hyderabad Commission are unable to see. There is not one tittle of evidence of any kind, still less of physiological proof, or paralysis of the heart in the case he describes. His whole statement on the subject is purely a conception of what he imagine occurs in these cases, and has no scientific value whatsoever."[35]

This last argument could equally well be applied to the Commission's conclusions about the accidental deaths of their animals. It is difficult to pardon the Commission for not attempting to investigate them, and to try and draw some scientific value from them. After all, its work was being done to shed light on the causes of death under chloroform, and so it is not unreasonable to expect that these deaths should have been investigated.

In 1902, Dr. E. H. Embley, of Melbourne in Australia, wrote at length of his careful research into the cause of death during chloroform anaesthesia.[36, 37, 38] He began by saying that clinical experience had, too frequently, been belittled whenever it did not coincide with the results of animal research. In England alone, out of 83 fatalities no less than 68 had occurred before the operations had begun. This early heart failure, Embley maintained, was nearly always sudden, and could happen even when the respiration was unimpaired. He, like others, pointed out that in 9 of the 154 dogs studied in Hyderabad death occurred early in the anaesthetic, and noted that these deaths were never investigated. The Commission had taken tracings only during the comparatively safe period when induction was over. Embley concluded that chloroform had both an immediate and a progressively paralytic effect on the heart, which seemed to be very sensitive to its actions, especially when a concentration greater than two per cent. was given. He concluded that chloroform concentrations not greater than one per cent. should be used during the early and dangerous induction phase of anaesthesia.

Embley's work, which had been done with the help of his colleague Professor Martin, was the subject of an enthusiastic editorial in the *British Medical Journal*.

"Previous work of a physiological kind can hardly be said to have settled the matter, for the number of opinions expressed regarding it is almost the same as the number of committees, commissions, and individual experimenters who have worked at it. In the majority of cases, however, the conclusions arrived at are contrary to those of the Hyderabad Commission, who looked upon respiratory failure as the primary cause of death; most of the other researchers look upon this as secondary to the failure in the circulatory apparatus. The Hyderabad Commission deserves much credit for pointing out the importance of watching the respiration during anaesthetization, and for indicating the most appropriate methods of administering the drug, but from the scientific point of view no impartial observer can maintain that they proved its main contention.

"Dr. Embley's contribution to the subject marks a distinct advance in knowledge, and we can heartily recommend our readers to peruse it carefully and study the numerous tracings by which he supports his conclusions. Dr. Embley is the anaesthetist at the Melbourne Hospital, and we understand that the impetus to his work was given by the occurrence of a number of unfortunate mishaps during the use of chloroform among the patients. The fact that such accidents have ceased since he has derived knowledge of their cause from his experiments is the best testimonial that can be adduced in favour of their value and trustworthiness. . . .

"A clinical observer would roughly divide the deaths he has witnessed from an anaesthetic into two main groups. There are those which occur during the later stages of the operation . . . [and] . . . those which occur in the induction or early period of chloroform anaesthesia, very often before the surgeon has touched the patient. It is these cases which have been the special object of study by Drs. Embley and Martin, and it is curious that in no previous piece of experimental work has this group of cases been investigated. The animal is usually anaesthetized in a box, and when it is fully under it is transferred for observation to the experimental table, but as Professor Martin put it . . . all the interesting things that occur in the box have been neglected. Dr. Embley . . . overcame the difficulty of observing the effects of the drug from the very commencement of its administration by preparing the animal sometime beforehand under the influence of another anaesthetic. The dosage of chloroform was estimated by a simple but very ingenious piece of apparatus, and the safe limit of the amount of chloroform vapour in the air was determined with accuracy."[39]

Predictably, Edward Lawrie entered a vigorous protest without delay.[40] He rounded on the Editor of the *British Medical Journal* for daring to bestow praise on Dr. Embley's research, the results of which he refuted completely. He ended by making his usual claim about the correctness of Syme's original views and the Hyderabad Commission's work.

Clearly nothing, but nothing, could have made Lawrie change his opinions. His absolute faith in Syme's totally fictitious arguments and, with considerably more justification, his own, large and successful experience made him didactic, obdurate, and intolerant. This habit of mind must have been fostered by his high position at Hyderabad where he remained in unchallenged authority for sixteen years. There, his was a superhuman task. He had to be a specialist in almost everything — the last court of appeal in virtually every branch of an expanding science. If nurses had to be trained he, with his wife (who had trained at The London Hospital), had to establish the training school and give many of the lectures and demonstrations as well. If medical students had to be made into doctors he had to do that too. His was the driving force at the Medical School and the Residency and Afzulgunj Hospitals. Primarily, he was a surgeon, judging by the amount of surgery he did, but he also assumed that he knew all there was to know about anaesthetics. In addition he was, no doubt, an ophthalmologist, a gynaecologist, obstetrician, pathologist, medico-legal expert, medical officer of health, and many more things besides. Such versatility was quite common in the nineteenth century, and was only made possible by the relative simplicity of medicine and surgery at the time. Even in medical schools situated in more advanced and less remote places than Hyderabad there were many men who held teaching appointments in two, or more, subjects. Lauder Brunton did so at Bart's.

Few of those who became drawn into the controversy first stirred up in January, 1889 at Hyderabad have emerged with any great credit. Those who opposed Lawrie and the Hyderabad Commission's views were, with the benefit of hindsight, correct, but they failed to press home the views that they held and, thereby, demolish Lawrie's zealous teachings. Nonetheless, by a process of attrition, the combined arguments of the many did, eventually, reduce the effects of Lawrie's extreme beliefs.

Lawrie's personal expertise with chloroform was unique and exemplary, but the majority of his writings on the subject were, at best, misguided and misleading and, at worst, cavalier and dangerous. Nonetheless, with the perspective of history, Edward Lawrie, wrong though he was, can be identified as one of the most influential participants in the frail speciality of Anaesthesia's first hundred years.

REFERENCES

[1] Sykes, W. S. (1960) *Essays on the First Hundred Years of Anaesthesia. Volume I.* Edinburgh: Livingstone.
[2] Hewitt, F. (1901) The teaching of anaesthetics. *Lancet*, **1**, 212–213.
[3] Lawrie, E. (1914) The position of chloroform. *British Medical Journal*, **1**, 623–624.
[4] Farquharson, R. (1914) The position of chloroform. *British Medical Journal*, **1**, 994–995.
[5] Lawrie, E. (1889) The Hyderabad Chloroform Commission. *Lancet*, **2**, 601.
[6] Brunton, T. L. (1898) An answer to Mr. Leonard Hill's rejoinder regarding the Hyderabad Commission. *British Medical Journal*, **1**, 1322–1324.
[7] Eastes, G. (1890) Relative safety of anaesthetics. *Lancet*, **1**, 823–824.
[8] Lawrie, E., Brunton, T. L., Bomford, G., & Hakim, R. D. (1890) Report of the Second Hyderabad Chloroform Commission. *Lancet*, **1**, 149–159.
[9] Lawrie, E. (1899) The Hyderabad Chloroform Commission. *Lancet*, **1**, 952–953.

[10] Lawrie, E. (1890) The Hyderabad Chloroform Commission. *Lancet*, **1**, 1389–1393.

[11] Lawrie, E. (1897) Partial anaesthesia with chloroform. *British Medical Journal*, **2**, 271–272.

[12] Lawrie, E. (1899) Notes on some cases illustrating the advantages of partial chloroform anaesthesia. *Lancet*, **1**, 1028–1029.

[13] Lawrie, E. The production of chloroform anaesthesia. *Lancet*, **1**, 1681–1682.

[14] Lawrie, E. (1901) *Chloroform: A manual for students and practitioners*. London: Churchill.

[14a] Brown, H. H. (1944) The Surgeon and the Anaesthetic. *British Medical Journal*, **2**, 191.

[15] Bellamy Gardner, H. (1901) The teaching of anaesthetics. *Lancet*, **1**, 1104–1105.

[16] Buxton, D. W. (1901) The teaching of anaesthetics. *Lancet*, **1**, 1105.

[17] Hewitt, F. W. (1901) The teaching of anaesthetics. *Lancet*, **1**, 1166–1167.

[18] Lawrie, E. (1894) Demonstration of the Hyderabad method of chloroform administration at The London Hospital, May 25th, 1894. *Lancet*, **1**, 1395–1396.

[19] Lawrie, E. (1907) Dr. Waller's address on the action of anaesthetics. *British Medical Journal*, **2**, 487.

[20] Lawrie, E. (1907) Dr. Waller's address on the action of anaesthetics. *British Medical Journal*, **2**, 555.

[21] Lawrie, E., Brunton, T. L., Bomford, G., & Hakim, R. D. (1890) Report of the Second Hyderabad Chloroform Commission, *Lancet*, **1**, 1140–1142.

[22] Brunton, T. L. (1890) An address on the experiments on anaesthetics conducted at Hyderabad. *British Medical Journal*, **1**, 347–350.

[23] Anonymous (1894) Discussion on chloroform. *British Medical Journal*, **2**, 14–16.

[24] Editorial (1888) *Lancet*, **2**, 523–524.

[25] Guthrie, L. G. (1894) On some fatal after-effects of chloroform on children. *Lancet*, **1**, 193–197.

[26] Guthrie, L. G. (1894) On some fatal after-effects of chloroform on children. *Lancet*, **1**, 257–261.

[27] Lawrie, E. (1914) The problem of chloroform. *British Medical Journal*, **1**, 995.

[28] Lawrie, E. (1903) The dosage of chloroform. *British Medical Journal*, **2**, 277–278.

[29] Leaf, C. H. (1892) Hyderabad Chloroform Commission. *British Medical Journal*, **2**, 327.

[30] Leaf, C. H. (1893) Experiments with chloroform and ether. *Lancet*, **1**, 988–991.

[31] Leaf, C. H. (1894) Deaths under chloroform. *Lancet*, **2**, 408–409.

[32] Stevenson, W. A. (1893) Chloroform anaesthesia. *Lancet*, **1**, 616.

[33] Mills, J. (1880) On watching the pulse during the administration of chloroform. *Lancet*, **2**, 912–913.

[34] Hill, L. (1897) The caustion of chloroform syncope. *British Medical Journal*, **1**, 957–962.

[35] Lawrie, E. (1897) Chloroform and the heart. *British Medical Journal*, **2**, 131–132.

[36] Embley, E. H. (1902) The causation of death during the administration of chloroform. *British Medical Journal*, **2**, 817–821.

[37] Embley, E. H. (1902) The causation of death during the administration of chloroform. *British Medical Journal*, **1**, 885–893.

[38] Embley, E. H. (1902) The causation of death during the administration of chloroform. *British Medical Journal*, **1**, 951–961.

[39] Editorial. (1902) The causation of death during the administration of chloroform. *British Medical Journal*, **1**, 975–976.

[40] Lawrie, E. (1902) The causation of death during the administration of chloroform. *British Medical Journal*, **1**, 1058.

CHAPTER 20

POSTSCRIPT

The lines of one of my favourite poems came vividly to my mind while I was working on the manuscript and notes left by the late Dr. Sykes on the Hyderabad Chloroform Commission and its various ramifications. They are, I think, especially appropriate to the life and actions of Edward Lawrie but, in some measure, can be applied to each of the principals mentioned in these essays, and also, with equal ease, to Stanley Sykes himself.

The final verse is an apt description, not only of historians themselves, but also of those whose actions they would describe, and of the vantage points from which they attempt their judgements.

When Earth's last picture is painted, and the tubes are twisted and dried,
When the oldest colours have faded, and the youngest critic has died,
We shall rest, and, faith, we shall need it — lie down for an aeon or two,
Till the Master of All Good Workmen shall put us to work anew.

And those that were good shall be happy: they shall sit in a golden chair;
They shall splash at a ten-league canvas with brushes of comets' hair.
They shall find real saints to draw from — Magdalene, Peter and Paul;
They shall work for an age at a sitting and never be tired at all!

And only the Master shall praise us, and only the Master shall blame;
And no one shall work for money, and no one shall work for fame,
But each for the joy of the working, and each, in his separate star,
Shall draw the Thing as he sees It for the God of Things as They are!

This poem is entitled *When Earth's last picture is painted* and was, appropriately enough, written by Rudyard Kipling in 1892.

INDEX